ITALIAN RECIPES 2022

MOUTH-WATERING AND EASY ANTIPASTI AND SOUPS

ANDREA LOI

ANDIAMO DA MANGIARE DA CARLO!

TABLE OF CONTENTS

Shrimp and Rice Salad 10

Shrimp, Orange, and Anchovy Salad 12

Sardine and Arugula Salad 14

Grilled Scallop Salad 17

Venetian Crab Salad 19

Calamari Salad with Arugula and Tomatoes 21

Lobster Salad 24

Tuscan Tuna and Bean Salad 27

Couscous Tuna Salad 29

Tuna Salad with Beans and Arugula 31

Friday-Night Tuna Salad 34

Gorgonzola and Hazelnut Dressing 37

Lemon Cream Dressing 38

Orange-Honey Dressing 39

Meat Broth 40

Chicken Broth 42

Antonietta's Bean Soup 44

Pasta and Beans 47

Creamy Bean Soup 49

Friulian Barley and Bean Soup 51

Bean and Mushroom Soup	53
Milan-Style Pasta and Beans	55
Lentil and Fennel Soup	59
Spinach, Lentil, and Rice Soup	61
Lentil and Greens Soup	63
Pureed Lentil Soup with Croutons	65
Chickpea Soup from Puglia	67
Chickpea and Pasta Soup	69
Ligurian Chickpea and Porcini Soup	71
Tuscan Bread and Vegetable Soup	74
Winter Squash Soup	78
"Cooked Water" Soup	80
Zucchini Pesto Soup	82
Leek, Tomato, and Bread Soup	84
Zucchini and Tomato Soup	86
Zucchini and Potato Soup	88
Creamy Fennel Soup	90
Mushroom and Potato Soup	92
Creamy Cauliflower Soup	94
Sicilian Tomato Barley Soup	96
Red Pepper Soup	98
Fontina, Bread, and Cabbage Soup	100

Creamy Mushroom Soup 102

Vegetable Soup with Pesto 104

Egg Soup from Pavia 106

Roman Egg Drop Soup 109

Egg Crepes in Broth 110

Semolina Fritters in Broth 111

Wafer Cookies 115

Sweet Ravioli 118

"Ugly-but-Good" Cookies 121

Double-Chocolate Nut Biscotti 123

Chocolate Kisses 126

No-Bake Chocolate "Salame" 129

Prato Biscuits 131

Umbrian Fruit and Nut Biscotti 133

Butter Rings 136

Lemon Knots 138

Spice Cookies 141

Wafer Cookies 143

Sweet Ravioli 146

"Ugly-but-Good" Cookies 149

Jam Spots 151

Double-Chocolate Nut Biscotti 153

Chocolate Kisses 156

No-Bake Chocolate "Salame" 159

Prato Biscuits 161

Umbrian Fruit and Nut Biscotti 163

Lemon Nut Biscotti 166

Walnut Biscotti 168

Almond Macaroons 170

Pine Nut Macaroons 173

Hazelnut Bars 175

Walnut Butter Cookies 177

Rainbow Cookies 179

Christmas Fig Cookies 183

Almond Brittle 187

Sicilian Nut Rolls 189

Sponge Cake 192

Citrus Sponge Cake 194

Lemon Olive-Oil Cake 197

Marble Cake 199

Rum Cake 202

Grandmother's Cake 205

Apricot Almond Cake 209

Summer Fruit Torte 212

Autumn Fruit Torte 214

Polenta and Pear Cake 216

FISH SALADS

Shrimp and Rice Salad

Insalata di Riso con Gamberi

Makes 4 servings

Fiumicino, outside of Rome, is best known as the location of one of Italy's largest airports, named for the artist Leonardo Da Vinci. But Fiumicino is also a seaport, where Romans like to go in the summer to enjoy the cool breezes and eat at one of the great seafood restaurants along the shore. At Bastianelli al Molo, we sat on the terrace under a big white umbrella and watched the sea. I had a multicourse meal that included this simple shrimp and rice salad.

Cooked long-grain rice hardens when it is refrigerated, so make this salad shortly before you plan to serve it.

2 cups long-grain rice

⅓ cup extra-virgin olive oil

3 tablespoons fresh lemon juice

1 pound medium shrimp, shelled and deveined

1 bunch arugula

2 medium tomatoes, cut into wedges

1. Bring 4 cups of water to a boil in a large saucepan. Add the rice and 1 teaspoon salt. Stir well. Reduce the heat to low, cover the pan, and cook until the rice is tender, 16 to 18 minutes. Pour the rice into a large serving bowl.

2. In a small bowl, whisk together the oil, lemon juice, and salt and pepper to taste. Stir half the dressing into the rice and let cool.

3. Trim the tough stems of the arugula and discard any yellowed or bruised leaves. Wash the arugula in several changes of cool water. Dry very well. Tear the arugula into bite-size pieces.

4. Bring 2 quarts of water to a boil in a medium saucepan. Add the shrimp and salt to taste. Bring to a simmer and cook until the shrimp are pink and just cooked through, about 2 minutes. Drain and cool under running water.

5. Cut the shrimp into bite-size pieces. Stir the shrimp and arugula into the rice. Add the rest of the dressing and stir well. Taste and adjust seasoning. Garnish with the tomatoes. Serve immediately.

Shrimp, Orange, and Anchovy Salad

Insalata di Gamberi, Arancia, e Acciughe

Makes 4 servings

One of my favorite Venetian restaurants is La Corte Sconta, "the hidden courtyard." Despite its name, it is not too difficult to find, as it is a very popular trattoria, serving a set menu of all seafood dishes. This salad, zesty with Dijon mustard, is inspired by one I ate there.

1 small red onion, thinly sliced

2 teaspoons Dijon mustard

1 garlic clove, lightly crushed

4 teaspoons fresh lemon juice

¼ cup extra-virgin olive oil

1 teaspoon chopped fresh rosemary

Salt and freshly ground black pepper

24 large shrimp, shelled and deveined

4 navel oranges, peeled, white pith removed and sliced

1 (2-ounce) can anchovy fillets, drained

1. Place the onion in a medium bowl with very cold water to cover. Let stand 10 minutes. Drain the onion and cover it again with very cold water and let stand 10 minutes more. (This will make the onion flavor less sharp.) Pat the onion dry.

2. In a large bowl, whisk together the mustard, garlic, lemon juice, oil, and rosemary with salt and freshly ground black pepper to taste.

3. Bring a medium saucepan of water to a boil over medium heat. Add the shrimp and salt to taste. Cook until the shrimp turn pink and are just cooked through, about 2 minutes, depending on their size. Drain and cool under running water.

4. Add the shrimp to the bowl with the dressing and toss well. Arrange the watercress on serving plates. Top with the orange slices. Spoon the shrimp and dressing over the oranges. Scatter the onion slices on top. Serve immediately.

Sardine and Arugula Salad

Insalata con le Sarde

Makes 2 servings

This salad is based on one I tasted in Rome that was served on top of a thick slice of toasted bread and served as bruschetta. Though I liked the combination, it was hard to eat. I prefer to serve the bread as an accompaniment. Canned sardines packed in olive oil have a delicious smoky flavor that adds a lot to this simple salad.

1 large bunch arugula

2 tablespoons olive oil

1 tablespoon fresh lemon juice

Salt and freshly ground black pepper

½ cup black cured olives, pitted and cut into 2 or 3 pieces

1 (3-ounce) can sardines in olive oil

2 green onions, cut into thin slices

4 slices Italian bread, toasted

1. Trim the tough stems of the arugula and discard any yellowed or bruised leaves. Wash the arugula in several changes of cool water. Dry very well. Tear the arugula into bite-size pieces.

2. In a large bowl, whisk together the oil, lemon juice, and salt and pepper to taste. Add the arugula, olives, sardines, and green onions and toss well. Taste and adjust seasoning.

3. Serve immediately with the toasted bread.

Grilled Scallop Salad

Insalata di Capesante alla Griglia

Makes 3 to 4 servings.

Large, plump sea scallops are delicious grilled and served on a bed of tender salad greens and tomatoes. The scallops can be cooked on an outside grill, but I make this salad all year round, so I cook the scallops most often on a grill pan. This salad is inspired by one I have enjoyed often at I Trulli Restaurant and Enoteca in New York.

Olive oil

1 pound large sea scallops, rinsed

2 tablespoons fresh lemon juice

Salt and freshly ground black pepper

2 tablespoons chopped fresh basil

1 tablespoon chopped fresh mint

2 large ripe tomatoes, cut into bite-size pieces

6 cups tender salad greens, torn into bite-size pieces

1. Heat a grill pan over medium-high heat until a drop of water sizzles when dropped on the surface. Brush the pan lightly with oil.

2. Pat the scallops dry and place them on the grill pan. Cook until the scallops are lightly browned, about 2 minutes. Turn the scallops and cook until browned and slightly translucent in the center, 1 to 2 minutes more.

3. In a large bowl, whisk together the lemon juice with 3 tablespoons oil. Add the scallops and toss well. Let stand 5 minutes, stirring once or twice.

4. Add the herbs and tomatoes to the scallops and stir gently.

5. Arrange the lettuce on serving plates. Top with the scallop mixture and serve immediately.

Venetian Crab Salad

Insalata di Granseola

Makes 6 servings

Venice has many wine bars, called bacari, *where people gather to meet friends and sample a glass of wine and small plates of food. This delicate salad made from large crabs called* granseole *is often served as a topping for crostini. In more formal restaurants, you will find it served elegantly in radicchio cups. It makes a nice starter for a summer meal.*

2 tablespoons chopped fresh flat-leaf parsley

¼ cup extra-virgin olive oil

2 tablespoons fresh lemon juice

Salt and freshly ground black pepper to taste

1 pound fresh crab meat, picked over

Radicchio leaves

1. In a medium bowl, whisk together the parsley, oil, lemon juice, and salt and pepper to taste. Add the crab meat and stir well. Taste for seasoning.

2. Arrange the radicchio leaves on serving plates. Scoop the salad onto the leaves. Serve immediately.

Calamari Salad with Arugula and Tomatoes

Insalata di Calamari

Makes 6 servings

The crisscross cuts on the surface of the calamari (squid) cause the pieces to curl up tightly as they cook. This not only tenderizes the calamari, but also makes it very attractive.

For best flavor, allow for good marinating time. You can prepare the calamari up to three hours ahead.

1½ pounds cleaned calamari (squid)

2 garlic cloves, minced

2 tablespoons chopped fresh flat-leaf parsley

5 tablespoons olive oil

2 tablespoons fresh lemon juice

Salt and freshly ground black pepper

1 large bunch arugula

1 tablespoon balsamic vinegar

1 cup cherry or grape tomatoes, halved

1. Slit the calamari lengthwise and open them flat. With a sharp knife, score the bodies, making diagonal lines about $1/4$-inch apart. Turn the knife and make diagonal lines in the opposite direction, forming a crisscross pattern. Cut each squid into 2-inch squares. Cut the base of each group of tentacles in half. Rinse and drain the pieces and put them in a bowl.

2. Add the garlic, parsley, 2 tablespoons of the olive oil, the lemon juice, and salt and pepper to taste, and toss well. Cover and marinate up to 3 hours ahead of cooking.

3. Transfer the squid and marinade into a large skillet. Cook over medium-high heat, stirring frequently, just until the squid are opaque, about 5 minutes.

4. Trim the tough stems of the arugula and discard any yellowed or bruised leaves. Wash the arugula in several changes of cool water. Dry very well. Tear the arugula into bite-size pieces. Arrange the arugula on a platter.

5. In a small bowl, whisk together the remaining 3 tablespoons oil and the vinegar, and salt and pepper to taste. Pour over the arugula and toss well. Spoon the squid over the arugula. Scatter the tomatoes on top and serve immediately.

Lobster Salad

Insalata di Aragosta

Makes 4 to 6 servings

Sardinia is famous for its shellfish, especially spiny lobsters, known as astice, *and sweet shrimp. My husband and I ate this fresh-tasting salad at a little seaside trattoria in Alghero as we watched the fishermen repairing their nets for the next day's work. One sat on the dock barefoot. With his toes, he clutched one end of the net and held it taut so that both of his hands were free for sewing.*

This salad could be a whole meal or a first course. A bottle of chilled Sardinian vernaccia would be the perfect accompaniment.

Some fish markets will steam the lobsters for you, saving you a step.

4 lobsters (about 1¼ pounds each)

1 medium red onion, halved and thinly sliced

6 basil leaves

4 tender celery ribs, thinly sliced

About ½ cup extra-virgin olive oil

2 to 3 tablespoons fresh lemon juice

Salt and freshly ground black pepper

Lettuce leaves

8 thin slices crusty Italian bread

1 garlic clove

3 large ripe tomatoes, cut into wedges

1. Place a rack or steamer basket in the bottom of a pot large enough to hold all four lobsters. (An 8- or 10-quart pot should work.) Add water to come just below the rack. Bring the water to a boil. Add the lobsters and cover the pot. When the water returns to a boil and steam escapes from the pot, cook the lobsters 10 minutes or longer, depending on their size. Transfer the lobsters to a platter and let cool.

2. Place the onion in a small bowl and cover with ice water. Let stand 15 minutes. Replace the water and let stand 15 minutes more. Drain and pat dry.

3. Meanwhile, remove the lobster meat from the shells. Break off the lobster tails. With poultry shears, remove the thin shell that covers the tail meat. Smack the claws with the blunt side of the

knife to crack them. Break the claws open. Remove the meat with your fingers. Cut the meat into thin slices and place it in a large bowl.

4. Stack the basil leaves and cut them crosswise into thin ribbons. Add the basil, celery, and onion to the bowl with the lobster. Drizzle with $1/4$ cup of the oil and the lemon juice, and sprinkle with salt and pepper to taste. Toss well. Arrange the lobster mixture on four plates lined with lettuce leaves.

5. Toast the bread, then rub it with a cut garlic clove. Drizzle the toast with the remaining oil and sprinkle with salt. Garnish the platter with the toast and tomato wedges. Serve immediately.

Tuscan Tuna and Bean Salad

Insalata di Tonno alla Toscana

Makes 6 servings

Tuscan cooks are famous for their ability to cook beans just right. Tender, creamy, and full of flavor, the beans elevate an ordinary dish into something special, such as this classic salad. If you can find it, buy ventresca di tonno, *tuna belly, canned in good olive oil. The belly is considered the finest part of the tuna. It is more expensive, but full of flavor, with a meaty texture.*

3 tablespoons extra-virgin olive oil

1 to 2 tablespoons fresh lemon juice

Salt and freshly ground black pepper

3 cups cooked or canned cannellini beans, drained

2 tender celery ribs, thinly sliced

1 small red onion, very thinly sliced

2 (7-ounce) cans Italian tuna packed in olive oil

2 or 3 Belgian endive, trimmed and separated into spears

1. In a medium bowl, whisk together the oil, lemon juice, and salt to taste and a generous grinding of pepper.

2. Add the beans, celery, onion, and tuna. Stir well.

3. Arrange the endive spears on a platter. Top with the salad. Serve immediately.

Couscous Tuna Salad

Insalata di Tonno e Cuscusu

Makes 4 servings

Couscous is eaten in several Italian regions, including parts of Sicily and Tuscany. Every year, the Sicilian town of San Vito lo Capo hosts a couscous festival that attracts hundreds of thousands of visitors from around the world. Traditionally, the couscous is cooked with a variety of seafood, meats, or vegetables and served hot. This quick tuna and couscous salad is a satisfying, modern dish.

1 cup quick-cooking couscous

Salt

2 tablespoons chopped fresh basil

3 tablespoons olive oil

2 tablespoons lemon juice

Freshly ground black pepper

1 (7-ounce) can Italian tuna packed in olive oil

2 tender celery ribs, chopped

1 tomato, chopped

1 small cucumber, peeled, seeded, and chopped

1. Cook the couscous with salt to taste, according to the package directions.

2. In a small bowl, whisk together the basil, oil, lemon juice, and salt and pepper to taste. Stir in the warm couscous. Mix well. Taste and adjust seasoning. Drain the tuna and place it in the bowl with the celery, tomato, and cucumber.

3. Stir well. Taste and adjust seasoning. Serve at room temperature or chill in the refrigerator briefly.

Tuna Salad with Beans and Arugula

Insalata di Tonno, Fagioli, e Rucola

Makes 2 to 4 servings

I think I could write a whole book about my favorite tuna salads. This is one I make often for a quick lunch or dinner.

1 large bunch arugula or watercress

2 cups cooked or canned cannellini or cranberry beans, drained

1 (7-ounce) can Italian tuna packed in olive oil

¼ cup chopped red onion

2 tablespoons capers, rinsed and drained

1 tablespoon fresh lemon juice

Salt and freshly ground black pepper

Lemon slices for garnish

1. Trim the tough stems of the arugula or watercress and discard any yellowed or bruised leaves. Wash the arugula in several changes of cool water. Dry very well. Tear the greens into bite-size pieces.

2. In a large salad bowl, stir together the beans, tuna and its oil, red onion, capers, and lemon juice. Toss well.

3. Stir in the greens and serve garnished with lemon slices.

Friday-Night Tuna Salad

Insalata di Venerdi Sera

Makes 4 servings

At one time, Fridays were meatless days in Catholic homes. Dinner at our house usually consisted of pasta and beans and this easy salad.

1 (7-ounce) can Italian tuna packed in olive oil

2 ribs celery with leaves, trimmed and sliced

2 medium tomatoes, cut into bite-size pieces

2 hard-cooked eggs, peeled and quartered

3 or 4 slices red onion, thinly sliced and quartered

Pinch of dried oregano

2 tablespoons extra-virgin olive oil

½ of a medium head of romaine lettuce, rinsed and dried

Lemon wedges

1. Place the tuna with its oil in a large bowl. Break the tuna into pieces with a fork.

2. Add the celery, tomatoes, eggs, and onion to the tuna. Sprinkle with the oregano and olive oil and toss lightly.

3. Arrange the lettuce leaves on a platter. Top with the tuna salad. Garnish with lemon wedges and serve immediately.

DRESSINGS

Gorgonzola and Hazelnut Dressing

Salsa di Gorgonzola e Nocciole

Makes about ⅔ cup

I had this dressing in Piedmont, where it was served on endive leaves, but it is good on any number of chewy greens, such as frisée, escarole, or spinach.

4 tablespoons extra-virgin olive oil

1 tablespoon red wine vinegar

Salt and freshly ground black pepper

2 tablespoons crumbled gorgonzola

¼ cup chopped toasted hazelnuts (see <u>How to Toast and Skin Nuts</u>)

In a small bowl, whisk together the oil, vinegar, and salt and pepper to taste. Stir in the gorgonzola and hazelnuts. Serve immediately.

Lemon Cream Dressing

Salsa di Limone alla Panna

Makes about ⅓ cup

A little bit of cream takes the edge off a lemony dressing. I like this on tender lettuce leaves.

3 tablespoons extra-virgin olive oil

1 tablespoon fresh lemon juice

1 tablespoon heavy cream

Salt and freshly ground black pepper

In a small bowl, whisk together all of the ingredients. Serve immediately.

Orange-Honey Dressing

Citronette al'Arancia

Makes about ⅓ cup

The sweetness of this dressing makes it a perfect match for mixed greens like mesclun. Or try it on a combination of watercress, red onions, and black olives.

3 tablespoons extra-virgin olive oil

1 teaspoon honey

2 tablespoons fresh orange juice

Salt and freshly ground black pepper

In a small bowl, whisk together all of the ingredients. Serve immediately.

Meat Broth

Brodo di Carne

Makes about 4 quarts

Here is a basic broth made from different kinds of meat to use for soups, risotti, and stews. A good broth should be full of flavor but not so aggressive that it takes over the flavor of the dish. Beef, veal, and poultry can be used, but avoid pork or lamb. Their flavor is strong and can overwhelm the broth. Vary the proportions of the meats for this broth to your own taste or according to the ingredients you have on hand.

2 pounds meaty beef bones

2 pounds veal shoulder with bones

2 pounds chicken or turkey parts

2 carrots, trimmed and cut into 3 or 4 pieces

2 celery ribs with leaves, cut into 3 or 4 pieces

2 medium onions, peeled but left whole

1 large tomato or 1 cup chopped canned tomatoes

1 garlic clove

3 or 4 sprigs fresh flat-leaf parsley with stems

1. In a large stockpot, combine the meat, bones, and chicken parts. Add 6 quarts cold water and bring to a simmer over medium heat.

2. Adjust the heat so that the water is barely simmering. Skim off the foam and fat that rises to the surface of the broth.

3. When the foam stops rising, add the remaining ingredients. Cook 3 hours, regulating the heat so that the liquid bubbles gently.

4. Let the broth cool briefly, then strain it into plastic storage containers. The broth can be used right away, or let it cool completely, then cover and store it in the refrigerator up to 3 days or in the freezer up to 3 months.

Chicken Broth

Brodo di Pollo

Makes about 4 quarts

An old chicken, known as a fowl, gives broth a fuller, richer flavor than a younger bird. If you can't find a fowl, try adding turkey wings or necks to the broth, but don't use too much turkey or the flavor will overwhelm the chicken.

After cooking, much of the flavor will be boiled out of the meat, but thrifty Italian cooks use it to make a salad or chop it up for a pasta or vegetable stuffing.

1 4-pound whole fowl or chicken

2 pounds chicken or turkey parts

2 celery ribs with leaves, cut up

2 carrots, cut up

2 medium onions, peeled and left whole

1 large tomato or 1 cup chopped canned tomatoes

1 garlic clove

3 or 4 sprigs fresh parsley

1. Place the fowl and chicken or turkey parts in a large stockpot. Add 5 quarts cold water and bring to a simmer over medium heat.

2. Adjust the heat so that the water is barely simmering. Skim off the foam and fat that rises to the surface of the broth.

3. Once the foam stops rising, add the remaining ingredients. Cook 2 hours, regulating the heat so that the liquid bubbles gently.

4. Let the broth cool briefly, then strain it into plastic storage containers. The broth can be used right away, or let it cool completely, then cover and store it in the refrigerator up to 3 days or in the freezer up to 3 months.

Antonietta's Bean Soup

Zuppa di Fagioli

Makes 8 servings

When I visited the Pasetti family's winery in Abruzzo, their cook, Antonietta, prepared this bean soup for lunch. It is based on the classic <u>Abruzzo-Style Ragù</u>, but you can use another tomato sauce with or without meat.

A food mill is used to smooth the beans and eliminate the skins. The soup can also be pureed in a food processor or blender. Antonietta served the soup with freshly grated Parmigiano-Reggiano, though she told us that it is traditional for diners in that region to season the soup with the seeds of a fresh green chile. Alongside the grated cheese, she passed around a plate with chiles and a knife, so that each diner could chop and add his or her own.

2 cups <u>Abruzzo-Style Ragù</u>, or another meat or tomato sauce

3 cups water

4 cups drained cooked dried or canned cranberry or cannellini beans

Salt and freshly ground black pepper to taste

4 ounces spaghetti, cut or broken into 2-inch pieces

Freshly grated Parmigiano-Reggiano

1 or 2 fresh green chiles, such as jalapeno (optional)

1. Prepare the ragù, if necessary. Then, in a large pot, combine the ragù and water. Pass the beans through a food mill into the pot. Cook over low heat, stirring occasionally, until the soup is hot. Add salt and pepper to taste.

2. Add the pasta and stir well. Cook, stirring often, until the pasta is soft. Add a little more water if the soup becomes too thick.

3. Serve hot or warm. Pass the cheese and fresh chiles, if using, separately.

Pasta and Beans

Pasta e Fagioli

Makes 8 servings

This Neapolitan version of bean and pasta soup (known by its dialect name as "pasta fazool") is typically served very thick, but it should still be eaten with a spoon.

¼ cup olive oil

2 celery ribs, chopped (about 1 cup)

2 garlic cloves, finely chopped

1 cup peeled, seeded, and chopped fresh tomatoes, or canned tomatoes

Pinch of crushed red pepper

Salt

3 cups drained cooked dried or canned cannellini or Great Northern beans

8 ounces ditalini or broken spaghetti

1. Pour the oil into a large saucepan. Add the celery and garlic. Cook, stirring frequently, over medium heat until the vegetables are tender and golden, about 10 minutes. Add the tomatoes, crushed red pepper, and salt to taste. Simmer until slightly thickened, about 10 minutes.

2. Add the beans to the tomato sauce. Bring the mixture to a simmer. Mash some of the beans with the back of a large spoon.

3. Bring a large pot of water to a boil. Add the salt to taste, then the pasta. Stir well. Cook over high heat, stirring frequently, until the pasta is tender, but slightly underdone. Drain the pasta, reserving some of the cooking water.

4. Stir the pasta into the bean mixture. Add a little of the cooking water, if needed, but the mixture should remain very thick. Turn off the heat and let stand about 10 minutes before serving.

Creamy Bean Soup

Crema di Fagioli

Makes 4 to 6 servings

I came upon a version of this recipe in A Tavola *("At the table"), an Italian cooking magazine. Creamy and smooth, this soup is pure, soothing comfort food.*

3 cups drained cooked dried or canned cannellini or Great Northern beans

About 2 cups homemade <u>Meat Broth</u> or a mix of half store-bought beef broth and half water

½ cup milk

2 egg yolks

½ cup freshly grated Parmigiano-Reggiano, plus more for serving

Salt and freshly ground black pepper

1. Puree the beans in a food processor, blender, or food mill.

2. In a medium saucepan, bring the broth to a simmer over medium heat. Stir in the bean puree and return to a simmer.

3. In a small bowl, beat together the milk and egg yolks. Pour about a cup of the soup into the bowl and whisk until smooth. Pour the mixture into the pot. Cook, stirring, until very hot but not boiling.

4. Stir in the Parmigiano-Reggiano and salt and pepper to taste. Serve hot with a sprinkle of additional cheese.

Friulian Barley and Bean Soup

Zuppa di Orzo e Fagioli

Makes 6 servings

Though it is better known in the United States as a small pasta shape, orzo *in Italian is the name for barley, one of the first grains ever cultivated. The region that is now Friuli in Italy was once part of Austria. The presence of barley reveals the Austrian roots of this soup.*

If using already cooked or canned beans, substitute 3 cups or two 16-ounce cans of drained beans, reduce the water to 4 cups, and cook the soup only 30 minutes in step 2. Then proceed as indicated.

2 tablespoons olive oil

2 ounces finely chopped pancetta

2 celery ribs, chopped

2 carrots, chopped

1 medium onion, chopped

1 garlic clove, finely chopped

1 cup (about 8 ounces) dried cannellini or <u>Great Northern beans</u>

½ cup pearl barley, rinsed and drained

Salt and freshly ground black pepper

1. Pour the oil into a large pot. Add the pancetta. Cook, stirring frequently, over medium heat until the pancetta is lightly browned, about 10 minutes. Add the celery, carrots, onion, and garlic. Cook, stirring frequently, until the vegetables are golden, about 10 minutes.

2. Add the beans and 8 cups water. Bring to a simmer. Cover and cook over low heat for $1^1/_2$ to 2 hours or until the beans are very tender.

3. Mash some of the beans with the back of a large spoon. Add the barley, and salt and pepper to taste. Cook 30 minutes or until the barley is tender. Stir the soup frequently so that the barley does not stick to the bottom of the pot. Add water if the soup is too thick. Serve hot or warm.

Bean and Mushroom Soup

Minestra di Fagioli e Funghi

Makes 8 servings

A chilly fall day in Tuscany had me craving a hearty bowl of soup and led me to a simple but memorable meal. At Il Prato, a restaurant in Pienza, the waiter announced that the kitchen had prepared a special bean soup that day. The soup was delicious, with an earthy, smoky flavor that I later learned came from the addition of dried porcini mushrooms. After the soup, I ordered some of the excellent pecorino cheese for which Pienza is famous.

½ ounce dried porcini mushrooms

1 cup warm water

2 medium carrots, chopped

1 celery rib, chopped

1 medium onion, chopped

1 cup peeled, seeded, and chopped fresh tomatoes or canned tomatoes

¼ cup chopped fresh flat-leaf parsley

6 cups homemade <u>Meat Broth</u> or <u>Chicken Broth</u> or a mix of half store-bought broth and half water

3 cups drained cooked dried or canned cannellini or great northern beans

½ cup medium-grain rice, such as Arborio

Salt and freshly ground black pepper to taste

1. Soak the mushrooms in the water for 30 minutes. Remove the mushrooms and reserve the liquid. Rinse the mushrooms under cold running water to remove any grit, paying special attention to the stems, where soil collects. Chop the mushrooms coarsely. Strain the mushroom liquid through a paper coffee filter into a bowl and reserve.

2. In a large pot, combine the mushrooms and their liquid, the carrots, celery, onion, tomato, parsley, and broth. Bring it to a simmer. Cook until the vegetables are tender, about 20 minutes.

3. Add the beans and rice and salt and pepper to taste. Cook until the rice is tender, 20 minutes, stirring occasionally. Serve hot or warm.

Milan-Style Pasta and Beans

Pasta e Fagioli alla Milanese

Makes 8 servings

Scraps of leftover fresh pasta, called maltagliati *("badly cut"), are typically used for this soup, or you could use fresh fettuccine cut into bite-size pieces.*

2 tablespoons unsalted butter

2 tablespoons olive oil

6 fresh sage leaves

1 tablespoon chopped fresh rosemary

4 carrots, chopped

4 celery ribs, chopped

3 medium boiling potatoes, chopped

2 onions, chopped

4 tomatoes, peeled, seeded, and chopped, or 2 cups chopped canned tomatoes

1 pound (about 2 cups) dried cranberry or cannellini beans (see <u>Country-Style Beans</u>) or 4 16-ounce cans

About 8 cups homemade <u>Meat Broth</u> or a mix of half store-bought beef or vegetable broth and half water

Salt and freshly ground black pepper

8 ounces fresh maltagliati, or fresh fettuccine cut into 1-inch pieces

Extra-virgin olive oil

1. In a large pot, melt the butter with the oil over medium heat. Stir in the sage and rosemary. Add the carrots, celery, potatoes, and onions. Cook, stirring often, until softened, about 10 minutes.

2. Stir in the tomatoes and beans. Add the broth and salt and pepper to taste. Bring the mixture to a simmer. Cook over low heat until all of the ingredients are very tender, about 1 hour.

3. Remove half of the soup from the pot and pass it through a food mill or puree it in a blender. Pour the puree back into the pot. Stir well and add the pasta. Bring the soup to a simmer, then turn off the heat.

4. Let the soup cool slightly before serving. Serve hot, with a drizzle of extra-virgin olive oil and a generous grinding of pepper.

Lentil and Fennel Soup

Zuppa di Lenticchie e Finocchio

Makes 8 servings

Lentils are one of the oldest legumes. They can be brown, green, red, or black, but in Italy the finest lentils are the tiny green ones from Castelluccio in Umbria. Unlike beans, lentils do not need to be soaked before cooking.

Save the feathery tops of the fennel to garnish the soup.

1 pound brown or green lentils, picked over and rinsed

2 medium onions, chopped

2 carrots, chopped

1 medium boiling potato, peeled and chopped

1 cup chopped fennel

1 cup fresh or canned tomatoes, chopped

¼ cup olive oil

Salt and freshly ground black pepper

1 cup tubetti, ditalini, or small shells

Fresh fennel tops, optional

Extra-virgin olive oil

1. In a large pot, combine the lentils, onions, carrots, potato, and fennel. Add cold water to cover by 1 inch. Bring the liquid to a simmer and cook over low heat 30 minutes.

2. Stir in the tomatoes and olive oil. Add salt and pepper to taste. Cook until the lentils are tender, about 20 minutes more. Add a little water as needed so that the lentils are just covered with the liquid.

3. Stir in the pasta and cook until the pasta is tender, 15 minutes more. Taste and adjust seasoning. Garnish with the chopped fennel tops, if available. Serve hot or warm, with a drizzle of extra-virgin olive oil.

Spinach, Lentil, and Rice Soup

Minestra di Lenticchie e Spinaci

Makes 8 servings

If less water is added and the rice is omitted, this soup becomes a side dish to serve with grilled fish fillets or pork. Escarole, kale, cabbage, Swiss chard, or other leafy greens can be used instead of the spinach.

1 pound lentils, picked over and rinsed

6 cups water

3 large garlic cloves, chopped

¼ cup extra-virgin olive oil

8 ounces spinach, stemmed and torn into bite-size pieces

Salt and freshly ground black pepper

1 cup cooked rice

1. In a large pot, combine the lentils, water, garlic, and oil. Bring to a simmer and cook over low heat 40 minutes. Add a little water as needed so that the lentils are just covered.

2. Stir in the spinach and the salt and pepper to taste. Cook until the lentils are tender, about 10 minutes more.

3. Add the rice and cook until heated through. Serve hot, with a drizzle of extra-virgin olive oil.

Lentil and Greens Soup

Minestra di Lenticchie e Verdura

Makes 6 servings

Look the lentils over before cooking them to eliminate any small stones or debris. For a heartier soup, add a cup or two of cooked ditalini or broken spaghetti.

¼ cup olive oil

1 medium onion, chopped

1 celery rib, chopped

1 medium carrot, chopped

2 garlic cloves, finely chopped

½ cup chopped canned Italian tomatoes

8 ounces lentils (about 1 cup), picked over and rinsed

Salt and freshly ground black pepper

1 pound escarole, spinach, or other leafy greens, trimmed and cut into bite-size pieces

½ cup freshly grated Pecorino Romano or Parmigiano-Reggiano

1. Pour the oil into a large pot. Add the onion, celery, carrot, and garlic and cook over medium heat for 10 minutes or until the vegetables are tender and golden. Stir in the tomatoes and cook 5 minutes more.

2. Add the lentils, salt and pepper, and 4 cups water. Bring the soup to a simmer and cook 45 minutes or until the lentils are tender.

3. Stir in the greens. Cover and cook 10 minutes, or until the greens are tender. Taste for seasoning.

4. Just before serving, stir in the cheese. Serve hot.

Pureed Lentil Soup with Croutons

Purèa di Lenticchie

Makes 6 to 8 servings

Crunchy slices of bread top this smooth lentil puree from Umbria. For added flavor, rub the croutons with a raw garlic clove while they are still warm.

1 pound lentils, picked over and rinsed

1 celery rib, chopped

1 carrot, chopped

1 large onion, chopped

1 large boiling potato, chopped

2 tablespoons tomato paste

Salt and freshly ground black pepper

2 tablespoons extra-virgin olive oil, plus more for serving

8 slices Italian or French bread

1. Place the lentils, vegetables, and tomato paste in a large pot. Add cold water to cover by 2 inches. Bring to a simmer. Cook 20 minutes. Add salt to taste and more water if needed to keep the ingredients covered. Cook 20 minutes more or until the lentils are very soft.

2. Drain the contents of the pot, reserving the liquid. Put the lentils and vegetables in a processor or blender and puree, in batches if necessary, until smooth. Pour the lentils back into the pot. Season to taste with salt and pepper. Reheat gently, adding some of the cooking liquid if needed.

3. In a large skillet, heat the 2 tablespoons olive oil over medium heat. Add the bread in a single layer. Cook until toasted and brown on the bottom, 3 to 4 minutes. Turn the bread pieces over and brown about 3 minutes more.

4. Remove the soup from the heat. Spoon into bowls. Top each bowl with a slice of toast. Serve hot, with a drizzle of olive oil

Chickpea Soup from Puglia

Minestra di Ceci

Makes 6 servings

In Puglia, this thick soup is made with short strips of fresh pasta known as lagane. *Fresh fettuccine cut into 3-inch strips can be substituted, as can small dried pasta shapes or broken spaghetti. Instead of a broth, anchovies are used to flavor this soup, with water as the cooking liquid. The anchovies melt into the soup and add a lot of character without being obvious.*

$\frac{1}{3}$ cup olive oil

3 garlic cloves, slightly crushed

2 2-inch sprigs fresh rosemary

4 anchovy fillets, chopped

$3\frac{1}{2}$ cups cooked chickpeas or 2 16-ounce cans, drained and liquid reserved

4 ounces fresh fettuccine, cut into 3-inch lengths

Freshly ground black pepper

1. Pour the oil into a large pot. Add the garlic and rosemary and cook over medium heat, pressing the garlic cloves with the back of a large spoon, until the garlic is golden, about 2 minutes. Remove and discard the garlic and rosemary. Add the anchovy fillets and cook, stirring, until the anchovy dissolves, about 3 minutes.

2. Add the chickpeas to the pot and stir well. Coarsely mash half of the chickpeas with the back of a spoon or a potato masher. Add just enough water or chickpea cooking liquid to cover the chickpeas. Bring the liquid to a simmer.

3. Stir in the pasta. Season to taste with a generous grind of black pepper. Cook until the pasta is tender yet firm to the bite. Remove from the heat and let stand 5 minutes. Serve hot, with a drizzle of extra-virgin olive oil.

Chickpea and Pasta Soup

Minestra di Ceci

Makes 6 to 8 servings

In the Marches region in central Italy, this soup sometimes is made with quadrucci, *small squares of fresh egg pasta. To make* quadrucci, *cut fresh fettuccine into short lengths to form small squares. Let each person drizzle his or her soup with a little extra-virgin olive oil.*

Of all legumes, I find chickpeas to be the trickiest to cook. Sometimes they take far longer to become tender than I expect. It is a good idea to prepare this soup in advance through step 2 and then reheat and finish it when ready to serve, to be sure the chickpeas have sufficient time to become tender.

1 pound dried chickpeas, soaked overnight (see Country-Style Beans)

¼ cup olive oil

1 medium onion, chopped

2 celery ribs, chopped

2 cups canned tomatoes, chopped

Salt

8 ounces ditalini or small elbows or shells

Freshly ground black pepper

Extra-virgin olive oil

1. Pour the oil into a large pot. Add the onion and celery and cook, stirring frequently, over medium heat for 10 minutes or until the vegetables are tender and golden. Add the tomatoes and bring to a simmer. Cook 10 minutes more.

2. Drain the chickpeas and add them to the pot. Add 1 teaspoon salt and cold water to cover by 1 inch. Bring to a simmer. Cook $1^1/_2$ to 2 hours or until the chickpeas are very tender. Add water if necessary to keep the chickpeas covered.

3. About 20 minutes before the chickpeas are done, bring a large pot of water to a boil. Add salt, then the pasta. Cook until the pasta is tender. Drain and add to the soup. Season to taste with salt and pepper. Serve hot, with a drizzle of extra-virgin olive oil.

Ligurian Chickpea and Porcini Soup

Pasta e Ceci con Porcini

Makes 4 servings

This is my version of a soup that is made in Liguria. Some cooks make it without the Swiss chard, while others include cardoons in the ingredients.

1/2 ounce dried porcini mushrooms

1 cup warm water

1/4 cup olive oil

2 ounces pancetta, chopped

1 medium onion, finely chopped

1 medium carrot, finely chopped

1 medium celery rib, finely chopped

1 garlic clove, finely chopped

3 cups cooked dried or drained canned chickpeas

8 ounces Swiss chard, cut crosswise into narrow strips

1 medium boiling potato, peeled and chopped

1 cup peeled, seeded, and chopped fresh or canned tomatoes

Salt and freshly ground black pepper

1 cup ditalini, tubetti, or other small pasta

1. Soak the mushrooms in the water for 30 minutes. Remove them and reserve the liquid. Rinse the mushrooms under cold running water to remove any grit. Chop them coarsely. Strain the liquid through a paper coffee filter into a bowl.

2. Pour the oil into a large pot. Add the pancetta, onion, carrot, celery, and garlic. Cook, stirring frequently, over medium heat until the onion and other aromatics are golden, about 10 minutes.

3. Stir in the chickpeas, Swiss chard, potato, tomatoes, and mushrooms with their liquid. Add water to just cover the ingredients, and salt and pepper to taste. Bring to a simmer and cook until the vegetables are tender and the soup is thickened, about 1 hour. Add water if the soup becomes too thick.

4. Stir in the pasta and 2 more cups water. Cook, stirring often, about 15 minutes, or until the pasta is tender. Let cool slightly before serving.

VEGETABLE SOUPS

Tuscan Bread and Vegetable Soup

Ribollita

Makes 8 servings

One summer in Tuscany, I was served this soup wherever I went, sometimes twice a day. I never tired of it, because every cook used her own combination of ingredients, and it was always good. This is really two recipes in one. The first is a mixed vegetable soup. The next day, the leftovers are reheated and mixed with day-old bread. The reheating gives the soup its Italian name, which means reboiled. This is typically done in the morning, and the soup is allowed to rest until lunchtime. Ribollita *is typically served warm or at room temperature, never steaming hot.*

Be sure to use a good-quality chewy Italian or country-style bread for the right texture.

4 cups homemade <u>Chicken Broth</u> or <u>Meat Broth</u> or a mix of half store-bought broth and half water

¼ cup olive oil

2 tender celery ribs, chopped

2 medium carrots, chopped

2 garlic cloves, finely chopped

1 small red onion, chopped

¼ cup chopped fresh flat-leaf parsley

1 tablespoon chopped fresh sage

1 tablespoon chopped fresh rosemary

1½ pounds peeled, seeded, and chopped fresh tomatoes or 1½ cups canned Italian peeled tomatoes with their juice, chopped

3 cups drained cooked dried or canned cannellini beans

2 medium boiling potatoes, peeled and diced

2 medium zucchini, chopped

1 pound cabbage or kale, thinly sliced (about 4 cups)

8 ounces green beans, trimmed and cut into bite-size pieces

Salt and freshly ground pepper to taste

About 8 ounces day-old Italian bread, thinly sliced

Extra-virgin olive oil

Very thin slices red onion (optional)

1. Prepare the broth, if necessary. Then, pour the olive oil into a large pot. Add the celery, carrots, garlic, onion, and herbs. Cook, stirring frequently, over medium heat until the celery and other aromatics are tender and golden, about 20 minutes. Add the tomatoes and cook 10 minutes.

2. Stir in the beans, remaining vegetables, and salt and pepper to taste. Add the broth and water to just cover. Bring to a simmer. Cook gently, over very low heat, until the vegetables are tender, about 2 hours. Let cool slightly, then if not using right away, store in the refrigerator overnight or up to 2 days.

3. When ready to serve, pour about 4 cups of the soup into a blender or food processor. Puree the soup, then transfer it to a pot along with the remaining soup. Reheat gently.

4. Choose a soup tureen or pot large enough to hold the bread and soup. Place a layer of bread slices on the bottom. Spoon on enough of the soup to cover the bread completely. Repeat the layering until all of soup is used and the bread is soaked. Let stand at least 20 minutes. It should be very thick.

5. Stir the soup to break up the bread. Drizzle with extra-virgin olive oil and sprinkle with the red onion. Serve warm or at room temperature.

Winter Squash Soup

Zuppa di Zucca

Makes 4 servings

At the fruttivendolo, *the fruit and vegetable market, Italian cooks can buy hunks of large pumpkins and other winter squashes to make this delicious soup. I generally use butternut or acorn squash. The crushed red pepper called* peperoncino *adds an unexpected piquancy.*

4 cups homemade <u>Chicken Broth</u> or a mix of half store-bought broth and half water

2 pounds winter squash, such as butternut or acorn

½ cup olive oil

2 garlic cloves, finely chopped

Pinch of crushed red pepper

Salt

¼ cup chopped fresh flat-leaf parsley

1. Prepare the broth if necessary. Then, peel the squash and remove the seeds. Cut into 1-inch pieces.

2. Pour the oil into a large pot. Add the garlic and crushed red pepper. Cook, stirring frequently, over medium heat until the garlic is lightly golden, about 2 minutes. Stir in the squash and salt to taste.

3. Add the broth and bring to a simmer. Cover and cook 35 minutes or until the squash is very soft.

4. With a slotted spoon, transfer the squash to a food processor or blender and puree until smooth. Return the puree to the pot with the broth. Bring the soup back to a simmer and cook 5 minutes. Add a little water if the soup is too thick.

5. Add salt to taste. Stir in the parsley. Serve hot.

"Cooked Water" Soup

Acquacotta

Makes 6 servings

Just a few vegetables, eggs, and leftover bread are needed to make this tasty Tuscan soup, so Italians jokingly call it "cooked water." Use whatever mushrooms are available.

¼ cup olive oil

2 celery ribs, thinly sliced

2 garlic cloves, chopped

1 pound assorted mushrooms, such as button, shiitake and cremini, trimmed and sliced

1 pound fresh plum tomatoes, peeled, seeded, and chopped, or 2 cups canned tomatoes

Pinch of crushed red pepper

6 eggs

6 slices Italian or French bread, toasted

4 to 6 tablespoons freshly grated pecorino cheese

1. Pour the oil into a medium pot. Add the celery and garlic. Cook, stirring frequently, over medium heat until softened, about 5 minutes.

2. Add the mushrooms and cook, stirring occasionally, until the mushroom juices evaporate. Add the tomatoes and the crushed red pepper and cook 20 minutes.

3. Add 4 cups water and salt to taste. Bring to a simmer. Cook 20 minutes more.

4. Just before serving, break one of the eggs into a cup. Carefully slip the egg into the hot soup. Repeat with the remaining eggs. Cover and cook over very low heat 3 minutes or until the eggs are done to taste.

5. Place a slice of toast in each serving bowl. Carefully ladle an egg on top and spoon on the hot soup. Sprinkle with the cheese and serve immediately.

Zucchini Pesto Soup

Zuppa di Zucchine al Pesto

Makes 4 to 6 servings

The aroma of the pesto when it is stirred into the hot soup is irresistible.

2 cups homemade <u>Chicken Broth</u> or a mix of half store-bought broth and half water

3 tablespoons olive oil

2 medium onions, chopped

4 small zucchini (about 1¼ pounds), scrubbed and chopped

3 medium boiling potatoes, peeled and chopped

Salt and freshly ground black pepper, to taste

1 cup broken spaghetti

Pesto

2 to 3 large garlic cloves

½ cup fresh basil

¼ cup fresh Italian flat-leaf parsley

½ cup grated Parmigiano-Reggiano, plus more for sprinkling

2 to 3 tablespoons extra-virgin olive oil

Salt and freshly ground black pepper

1. Prepare the broth, if necessary. Then, pour the oil into a medium pot. Add the onions. Cook, stirring often, over medium heat until the onions are tender and golden, about 10 minutes. Add the zucchini and potatoes and cook, stirring occasionally, 10 minutes. Add the chicken broth and 4 cups water. Bring the liquid to a simmer and cook 30 minutes. Add salt and pepper to taste.

2. Stir in the pasta. Simmer 15 minutes more.

3. Prepare the pesto: In a food processor, chop the garlic, basil, and parsley until very fine. Add the cheese and gradually drizzle in the olive oil to make a thick paste. Season to taste with salt and pepper.

4. Transfer the pesto to a medium bowl; with a whisk, beat about 1 cup of the hot soup into the pesto. Stir the mixture into the pot with the remaining soup. Let rest 5 minutes. Taste and adjust seasoning. Serve with additional cheese.

Leek, Tomato, and Bread Soup

Pappa al Pomodoro

Makes 4 to servings

Tuscans eat a lot of soup and make many of them with bread instead of pasta or rice. This is one that is a favorite in the early fall when there are plenty of ripe tomatoes and fresh leeks around. It is also good in the winter, made with canned tomatoes.

6 cups homemade Chicken Broth or a mix of half store-bought broth and half water

3 tablespoons olive oil, plus more for drizzling

2 medium leeks

3 large garlic cloves

Pinch of crushed red pepper

2 cups peeled, seeded, and chopped fresh tomatoes, or canned tomatoes

Salt

½ loaf day-old Italian whole-wheat bread, cut into 1-inch cubes (about 4 cups)

½ cup torn fresh basil

Extra-virgin olive oil

1. Prepare the broth, if necessary. Then, trim off the roots and dark green portion of the leeks. Cut the leeks in half lengthwise and rinse thoroughly under cool running water. Chop fine.

2. Pour the oil into a large pot. Add the leeks and cook, stirring frequently, over medium-low heat until softened, about 5 minutes. Stir in the garlic and crushed red pepper.

3. Add the tomatoes and broth and bring to a simmer. Cook 15 minutes, stirring occasionally. Add salt to taste.

4. Stir the bread into the soup and cook 20 minutes, stirring occasionally. The soup should be thick. Add more bread if necessary.

5. Remove from the heat. Stir in the basil and let stand 10 minutes. Serve hot, with a drizzle of extra-virgin olive oil.

Zucchini and Tomato Soup

Zuppa di Zucchine e Pomodori

Makes 6 servings

Though small zucchini have better flavor, even larger vegetables are good in this soup, because their wateriness and lack of flavor are not noticeable with all of the other flavorful ingredients.

5 cups homemade <u>Chicken Broth</u> or a mix of half store-bought broth and half water

3 tablespoons olive oil

1 medium onion, finely chopped

1 garlic clove, chopped

1 teaspooon chopped fresh rosemary

1 teaspoon chopped fresh sage

1½ cups peeled, seeded, and chopped tomatoes

1½ pounds zucchini, chopped

Salt and freshly ground black pepper

3 cups day-old Italian or French bread cubes

Freshly grated Parmigiano-Reggiano

1. Prepare the broth, if necessary. Then, pour the oil into a large pot. Add the onion, garlic, rosemary, and sage. Cook over medium heat, stirring frequently, until the onion is golden, about 10 minutes.

2. Add the tomatoes and stir well. Add the broth and bring to a simmer. Stir in the zucchini and cook 30 minutes or until tender. Season to taste with salt and pepper.

3. Stir in the bread cubes. Cook until the bread is soft, about 10 minutes. Let rest 10 minutes more before serving. Serve with grated Parmigiano-Reggiano.

Zucchini and Potato Soup

Minestra di Zucchine e Patate

Makes 4 servings

This soup is typical of what you might be served in summertime at homes throughout southern Italy. Feel free to change it as an Italian cook would, switching the zucchini for another vegetable such as green beans, tomatoes, or spinach and substituting basil or mint for the parsley.

6 cups homemade <u>Chicken Broth</u> or a mix of half store-bought broth and half water

2 tablespoons olive oil

1 medium onion, finely chopped

1 pound boiling potatoes (about 3 medium), peeled and chopped

1 pound zucchini (about 4 small), scrubbed and chopped

Salt and freshly ground black pepper

2 tablespoons chopped flat-leaf parsley

Freshly grated Parmigiano-Reggiano or Pecorino Romano

1. Prepare the broth, if necessary. Then, pour the oil into a medium pot. Add the onion and cook, stirring frequently, over medium heat until tender and golden, about 10 minutes.

2. Stir in the potatoes and zucchini. Add the broth and salt and pepper to taste. Bring to a simmer and cook until the vegetables are tender, about 30 minutes.

3. Add salt and pepper to taste. Stir in the parsley. Serve with the grated cheese.

Creamy Fennel Soup

Zuppa di Finocchio

Makes 6 servings

Potatoes and fennel have an affinity for each other. Serve this soup garnished with chopped fennel leaves and a drizzle of extra-virgin olive oil.

6 cups homemade <u>Chicken Broth</u> or a mix of half store-bought broth and half water

2 large leeks, trimmed

3 medium fennel bulbs (about 2½ pounds)

2 tablespoons unsalted butter

1 tablespoon olive oil

5 boiling potatoes, peeled and sliced

Salt and freshly ground black pepper

Extra-virgin olive oil

1. Prepare the broth, if necessary. Then, cut the leeks in half lengthwise and rinse them well to eliminate all traces of sand between the layers. Chop coarsely.

2. Trim the fennel stalks even with the bulbs, reserving some of the feathery green leaves for a garnish. Trim away the base and any brown spots. Cut the bulbs into thin slices.

3. In a large pot, melt the butter with the oil over medium heat. Add the leeks and cook until soft, about 10 minutes. Add the fennel, potatoes, broth, and salt and pepper to taste. Bring to a simmer and cook until the vegetables are very soft, about 1 hour.

4. With a slotted spoon, transfer the vegetables to a food processor or blender. Process or blend until smooth.

5. Return the vegetables to the pot and reheat gently. Spoon into soup bowls, sprinkle with the reserved fennel tops, and drizzle with olive oil. Serve hot.

Mushroom and Potato Soup

Minestra di Funghi e Patate

Makes 6 servings

Here is another soup from Friuli-Venezia Giulia, a region renowned for excellent mushrooms. Fresh porcini mushrooms would be used there, but because they are hard to find, I substitute a combination of wild and cultivated mushrooms. Both potatoes and barley are added as thickeners.

8 cups homemade <u>Meat Broth</u> or a mix of half store-bought broth and half water

2 tablespoons olive oil

2 ounces sliced pancetta, finely chopped

1 medium onion, finely chopped

2 celery ribs, finely chopped

1 pound assorted mushrooms, such as white, cremini, and portabello

4 tablespoons chopped fresh flat-leaf parsley

2 garlic cloves, finely chopped

3 medium boiling potatoes, peeled and chopped

Salt and freshly ground black pepper

½ cup pearl barley

1. Prepare the broth, if necessary. Pour the oil into a large pot. Add the pancetta. Cook, stirring frequently, over medium heat until golden, about 10 minutes. Add the onion and celery and cook, stirring occasionally, until softened, about 5 minutes.

2. Add the mushrooms, 2 tablespoons of the parsley, and the garlic. Cook, stirring often, until the mushroom juices evaporate, about 10 minutes.

3. Stir in the potatoes, salt, and pepper. Add the broth and bring to a simmer. Add the barley and cook, uncovered, over low heat for 1 hour or until the barley is tender and the soup is thickened.

4. Sprinkle with the remaining parsley and serve hot.

Creamy Cauliflower Soup

Vellutata di Cavolfiore

Makes 6 servings

An elegant soup to serve at the start of a special dinner. If you have some truffle oil or paste, try adding a little to the soup just before serving, leaving out the cheese.

1 medium cauliflower, trimmed and cut into 1-inch florets

Salt

3 tablespoons unsalted butter

¼ cup all-purpose flour

About 2 cups milk

Freshly grated nutmeg

½ cup heavy cream

¼ cup freshly grated Parmigiano-Reggiano

1. Bring a large pot of water to a boil. Add the cauliflower and salt to taste. Cook until the cauliflower is very tender, about 10 minutes. Drain well.

2. In a medium saucepan, melt the butter over medium heat. Add the flour and stir well for 2 minutes. Very slowly stir in 2 cups milk and salt to taste. Bring to a simmer and cook 1 minute, stirring constantly, until thickened and smooth. Remove from the heat. Stir in the nutmeg and cream.

3. Transfer the cauliflower to a food processor or blender. Puree, adding a little of the sauce, if necessary, to make the puree smooth. Transfer the puree to the pan with the remaining sauce. Stir well. Heat gently, adding more milk if necessary to make a thick soup.

4. Remove from the heat. Taste and adjust seasoning. Stir in the cheese and serve.

Sicilian Tomato Barley Soup

Minestra d'Orzo alla Siciliana

Makes 4 to 6 servings

Rather than grate the cheese, Sicilians often serve soup with cheese chopped into small bits. It never fully melts into the soup, and you can taste some of the cheese in each bite.

8 cups homemade <u>Chicken Broth</u> or <u>Meat Broth</u> or a mix of half store-bought broth and half water

8 ounces pearl barley, picked over and rinsed

2 medium tomatoes, peeled, seeded, and chopped, or 1 cup chopped canned tomatoes

1 celery rib, finely chopped

1 medium onion, finely chopped

Salt and freshly ground black pepper

1 cup diced Pecorino Romano

1. Prepare the broth, if necessary. In a large pot, combine the broth, barley, and vegetables and bring to a simmer. Cook until the barley is tender, about 1 hour. Add water if the soup becomes too thick.

2. Season with salt and pepper to taste. Spoon the soup into bowls, scattering the cheese over the top.

Red Pepper Soup

Zuppa di Peperoni Rossi

Makes 6 servings

The vibrant red-orange color of this soup is an appealing and appropriate cue to the refreshing, delicious flavor. It is inspired by a soup I tasted at Il Cibreo, a popular trattoria in Florence. I like to serve it with warm focaccia.

6 cups homemade <u>Chicken Broth</u> or a mix of half store-bought broth and half water

2 tablespoons olive oil

1 medium onion, chopped

1 celery rib, chopped

1 carrot, chopped

5 large red bell peppers, seeded and chopped

5 medium boiling potatoes, peeled and chopped

2 tomatoes, cored and chopped

Salt and freshly ground black pepper

1 cup milk

Freshly grated Parmigiano-Reggiano

1. Prepare the broth, if necessary. Then, pour the oil into a large pot. Add the onion, celery, and carrot. Cook, stirring frequently, over medium heat until the vegetables are tender and golden, about 10 minutes.

2. Add the peppers, potatoes, and tomatoes and stir well. Add the broth and bring to a simmer. Lower the heat and cook 30 minutes or until the vegetables are very tender.

3. With a slotted spoon, transfer the vegetables to a food processor or blender. Puree until smooth.

4. Pour the vegetable puree into the pot. Heat the soup gently and stir in the milk. Do not allow the soup to boil. Add salt and pepper to taste. Serve hot, sprinkled with cheese.

Fontina, Bread, and Cabbage Soup

Zuppa alla Valpelline

Makes 6 servings

One of my fondest memories of the Valle d'Aosta is the aromatic fontina cheese and flavorful whole grain bread of the region. The cheese is made from cows' milk and aged in mountain caves. Look for a cheese with a natural rind and the silhouette of a mountain pressed into the top to be sure you are getting the real fontina. Use a good, chewy bread for this hearty soup. Crinkly Savoy cabbage is milder tasting than the smooth-leaf variety.

8 cups homemade <u>Meat Broth</u> or a mix of half store-bought beef broth and half water

2 tablespoons unsalted butter

1 small Savoy cabbage, thinly shredded

Salt

¼ teaspoon freshly ground nutmeg

¼ teaspoon ground cinnamon

Freshly ground black pepper

12 ounces Fontina Valle d'Aosta

12 slices crusty seedless rye, pumpernickel, or whole-wheat bread, toasted

1. Prepare the broth, if necessary. Then, melt the butter in a large pot. Add the cabbage and salt to taste. Cover and cook on low heat for 30 minutes, stirring occasionally, until the cabbage is tender.

2. Preheat the oven to 350°F. Put the broth, nutmeg, cinnamon, salt, and pepper in a large pot and bring to a simmer over medium heat.

3. Place 4 slices of bread in the bottom of a deep 3-quart ovenproof Dutch oven or deep, heavy pot or baking dish. Cover with half of the cabbage and one third of the cheese. Repeat with another layer of bread, cabbage, and cheese. Top with the remaining bread. Carefully pour on the hot broth. Tear the reserved cheese into bits and scatter it on top of the soup.

4. Bake the casserole until browned and bubbling, about 45 minutes. Let rest 5 minutes before serving.

Creamy Mushroom Soup

Zuppa di Funghi

Makes 8 servings

Thanksgiving is not a holiday celebrated in Italy, but I often serve this creamy fresh and dried mushroom soup from northern Italy as part of my holiday menu.

8 cups homemade <u>Meat Broth</u> or a mix of half store-bought beef broth and half water

1 ounce dried porcini mushrooms

2 cups hot water

2 tablespoons unsalted butter

1 medium onion, finely chopped

1 garlic clove, finely chopped

1 pound white mushrooms, thinly sliced

½ cup dry white wine

1 tablespoon tomato paste

½ cup heavy cream

Chopped fresh flat-leaf parsley, for garnish

Salt and freshly ground black pepper

1. Prepare the broth, if necessary. Then, put the porcini mushrooms in the water and let soak 30 minutes. Remove the mushrooms from the bowl and reserve the liquid. Rinse the mushrooms under cold running water to removing any grit, paying special attention to the ends of the stems where soil collects. Chop the mushrooms coarsely. Strain the mushroom liquid through a paper coffee filter into a bowl.

2. In a large pot, melt the butter over medium heat. Add the onion and garlic and cook 5 minutes. Stir in all of the mushrooms and cook, stirring occasionally, until the mushrooms turn lightly golden, about 10 minutes. Add salt and pepper to taste.

3. Add the wine and bring to a simmer. Stir in the broth, mushroom liquid, and tomato paste. Lower the heat and simmer 30 minutes.

4. Stir in the cream. Sprinkle with parsley and serve immediately.

Vegetable Soup with Pesto

Minestrone al Pesto

Makes 6 to 8 servings

In Liguria, a dollop of fragrant pesto sauce is added to bowls of minestrone. It is not essential, but it really lifts the flavor of the soup.

¼ cup olive oil

1 medium onion, chopped

2 carrots, chopped

2 celery ribs, chopped

4 ripe tomatoes, peeled, seeded, and chopped

1 pound Swiss chard or spinach, chopped

3 medium boiling potatoes, peeled and chopped

3 small zucchini, chopped

8 ounces green beans, cut into ½-inch pieces

8 ounces shelled fresh cannellini or borlotti beans or 2 cups drained cooked dried or canned beans

Salt and freshly ground black pepper

1 recipe <u>Pesto</u>

4 ounces small pasta shapes such as tubetti or elbows

1. Pour the oil into a large pot. Add the onions, carrots, and celery. Cook, stirring frequently, over medium heat until the vegetables are tender and golden, about 10 minutes.

2. Stir in the tomatoes, chard, potatoes, zucchini, and beans. Add enough water to just cover the vegetables. Add salt and pepper to taste. Cook, stirring from time to time, until the soup is thickened and the vegetables are soft, about 1 hour. Add a little water if it becomes too thick.

3. Meanwhile, prepare the pesto, if necessary. When the soup has thickened, add the pasta. Cook, stirring, until the pasta is tender, about 10 minutes. Let cool slightly. Serve hot, passing a bowl of the pesto, to be added at the table, or ladle the soup into bowls and dollop some pesto in the center of each.

Egg Soup from Pavia

Zuppa alla Pavese

Makes 4 servings

Eggs poached in broth are a quick and delicious meal. The soup is ready to serve when the whites are just set and the yolks are still soft.

2 quarts homemade <u>Meat Broth</u> or a mix of half store-bought broth and half water

4 slices country bread, lightly toasted

4 large eggs, at room temperature

4 to 6 tablespoons freshly grated Parmigiano-Reggiano

Salt and freshly ground black pepper

1. Prepare the broth, if necessary. If not freshly made, heat the broth to a simmer. Season to taste with salt and pepper.

2. Have ready 4 heated soup bowls. Place a slice of toast in each bowl, then crack an egg over each slice of toast.

3. Pour the hot broth over the eggs to cover by a few inches. Sprinkle with the cheese. Let stand until the egg white is cooked to taste. Serve hot.

Roman Egg Drop Soup

Stracciatella

Makes 4 servings

Stracciatella *means "little rags," a reference to the appearance of the eggs in the soup. To enhance the flavor of the broth, you can add a little lemon juice or ground nutmeg.*

8 cups homemade <u>Chicken Broth</u> or a mix of half store-bought broth and half water

3 large eggs

¼ cup freshly grated Parmigiano-Reggiano

Salt and freshly ground black pepper

1 tablespoon very finely chopped fresh flat-leaf parsley

1. Prepare the broth, if necessary. If not freshly made, heat the broth until it is simmering.

2. In a small bowl, beat the eggs, cheese, salt, and pepper until well blended. Slowly pour the mixture into the broth, stirring constantly with a fork, just until the eggs are set and form ribbons. Stir in the parsley and serve immediately.

Egg Crepes in Broth

Scrippelle 'mbusse

Makes 6 servings

Scrippele *is Abruzzese dialect for* crespelle, *or crepes. These are the same crepes that are layered with cheese, mushrooms, and tomato sauce in the* Abruzzese Crepe and Mushroom Timbale *recipe. Here, they are filled with grated cheese and served in broth.*

8 cups homemade Chicken Broth or a mix of half store-bought broth and half water

12 Crepes

½ cup freshly grated Parmigiano-Reggiano

2 tablespoons finely chopped fresh Italian flat-leaf parsley

1. Prepare the broth, if necessary. Then, prepare the crepes, if necessary. Sprinkle each crepe with some of the cheese and parsley. Roll up the crepes to form tubes. Have ready 6 heated soup bowls. Place 2 tubes in each bowl.

2. If not hot, heat the broth until simmering. Spoon the hot broth onto the crepe tubes and serve immediately.

Semolina Fritters in Broth

Frittatine di Semola in Brodo

Makes 6 servings

At a formal dinner party at an elegant New York Italian restaurant, I got to talking with my friend Tony Mazzola about the foods we enjoyed as children. Tony told me about the simple soup his mother, Lydia, who came from Sicily, used to serve. As we ate our guinea hen and risotto covered in rare and expensive white truffles matched with fine wines, he described this comforting soup of tasty little semolina and cheese fritters in chicken broth. His mother only served it around Christmas and the New Year because, she said, its simplicity was good for you after all the rich food eaten during the holidays. A few days later, the fancy meal was all but forgotten, but I couldn't wait to try Tony's soup. This is the recipe as he and his sister Emilia were able to recreate it.

Note that the skillet is brushed very lightly with olive oil before the fritters are fried. There is no need to use more. The fritters brown and hold their shape better with less oil.

6 cups homemade <u>Chicken Broth</u> or a mix of half store-bought broth and half water

2½ cups water

1 teaspoon salt

1 cup fine ground semolina

1 large egg, beaten

1 cup freshly grated Parmigiano-Reggiano

2 tablespoons chopped fresh flat-leaf parsley

Freshly ground black pepper

Olive oil

1. Prepare the broth, if necessary. Then, in a medium saucepan over medium heat, bring the water to a simmer. Whisk in the semolina and salt. Reduce the heat to low and cook, stirring, until the semolina is thickened, about 2 minutes.

2. Remove the pot from the heat. Whisk in the egg, cheese, parsley, and pepper to taste.

3. Line a tray with a piece of plastic wrap. Scrape the semolina mixture onto the plastic and spread it out to a ½-inch thickness. Let cool to room temperature, at least 30 minutes. Use

immediately or cover with plastic wrap and store in the refrigerator up to 24 hours.

4. Just before serving the soup, cut the semolina mixture into bite-size pieces. Brush a large non-stick skillet with olive oil and heat the skillet over medium heat. Add enough of the semolina pieces as will fit comfortably in one layer without crowding. Cook until golden brown, about 4 to 5 minutes. Turn the pieces and brown the other side, about 4 to 5 minutes more. Remove the pieces to a plate. Cover with foil and keep warm. Brown the remaining semolina pieces in the same way.

5. Meanwhile, bring the broth to a simmer. Divide the semolina fritters among 4 bowls. Spoon on the broth. Serve immediately.

DESSERTS

Wafer Cookies

Pizzelle

Makes about 2 dozen

Many families in central and southern Italy are proud of their pizzelle irons, beautifully crafted forms traditionally used to make these pretty wafers. Some irons are embossed with the original owner's initials, while others have silhouettes such as a couple toasting each other with a glass of wine. They were once a typical wedding gift.

Though charming, these old fashioned irons are heavy and unwieldy on today's stoves. An electric pizzelle press, similar to a waffle iron, does an efficient and quick job of turning out these cookies.

When they are freshly made, pizzelle are pliable and can be molded into cone, tube, or cup shapes. They can be filled with whipped cream, ice cream, cannoli cream, or fruit. They cool and crisp in no time, so you must work quickly and carefully to shape them. Of course, they are good flat as well.

1¾ cups unbleached all-purpose flour

1 teaspoon baking powder

Pinch of salt

3 large eggs

⅔ cup sugar

1 tablespoon pure vanilla extract

1 stick (½ cup) unsalted butter, melted and cooled

1. Preheat the pizzelle maker according to the manufacturer's directions. In a bowl, stir together the flour, baking powder, and salt.

2. In a large bowl, beat the eggs, sugar, and vanilla with an electric mixer on medium speed until thick and light, about 4 minutes. Beat in the butter. Stir in the dry ingredients until just blended, about 1 minute.

3. Place about 1 tablespoon of the batter in the center of each pizzelle mold. (The exact amount will depend on the design of the mold.) Close the cover and bake until lightly golden. This will depend on the maker and how long the mold has been heating. Check it carefully after 30 seconds.

4. When the pizzelle are golden, slide them off the molds with a wooden or plastic spatula. Let cool flat on a wire rack. Or, to

make cookie cups, bend each pizzelle into the curve of a wide coffee or dessert cup. To make cannoli shells, shape them around cannoli tubes or a wooden dowel.

5. When the pizzelle are cool and crisp, store them in an airtight container until ready to use. These last for several weeks.

Variation: *Anise*: Substitute 1 tablespoon anise extract and 1 tablespoon anise seeds for the vanilla. *Orange or Lemon*: Add 1 tablespoon grated fresh orange or lemon zest to the egg mixture. *Rum or Almond*: Stir in 1 tablespoon rum or almond extract instead of the vanilla. *Nut*: Stir in $1/4$ cup of nuts ground to a very fine powder along with the flour.

Sweet Ravioli

Ravioli Dolci

Makes 2 dozen

Jam fills these crisp dessert ravioli. Any flavor will do, as long as it has a thick consistency so that it will stay in place and not ooze out of the dough as it bakes. This was a favorite recipe of my father, who perfected it from his memories of the cookies his mother used to make.

1¾ cup all-purpose flour

½ cup potato or corn starch

½ teaspoon salt

½ cup (1 stick) unsalted butter, at room temperature

½ cup sugar

1 large egg

2 tablespoons rum or brandy

1 teaspoon grated lemon zest

1 teaspoon pure vanilla extract

1 cup thick sour cherry, raspberry, or apricot jam

1. In a large bowl, sift together the flour, starch, and salt.

2. In a large bowl with an electric mixer, beat the butter with the sugar until light and fluffy, about 2 minutes. Beat in the egg, rum, zest, and vanilla. On low speed, stir in the dry ingredients.

3. Divide the dough in half. Shape each half into a disk. Wrap each separately in plastic and refrigerate 1 hour up to overnight.

4. Preheat the oven to 350°F. Grease 2 large baking sheets.

5. Roll out the dough to a $1/8$-inch thickness. With a fluted pastry or pasta cutter, cut the dough into 2-inch squares. Arrange the squares about 1 inch apart on the prepared baking sheets. Place $1/2$ teaspoon of the jam in the center of each square. (Do not use more jam, or the filling will leak out as it bakes.)

6. Roll out the remaining dough to a $1/8$-inch thickness. Cut the dough into 2-inch squares.

7. Cover the jam with the dough squares. Press the edges all around with a fork to seal in the filling.

8. Bake 16 to 18 minutes, or until lightly browned. Have ready 2 wire cooling racks.

9. Transfer the baking sheets to the racks. Let the cookies cool 5 minutes on the baking sheets, then transfer them to the wire racks to cool completely. Sprinkle with confectioner's sugar. Store in an airtight container up to 1 week.

"Ugly-but-Good" Cookies

Brutti ma Buoni

Makes 2 dozen

"Ugly but good" is the meaning of the name of these Piedmontese cookies. The name is only half-true: The cookies are not ugly, but they are good. The technique for making these is unusual. The cookie batter is cooked in a saucepan before it is baked.

3 large egg whites, at room temperature

Pinch of salt

1½ cups sugar

1 cup unsweetened cocoa powder

1¼ cups hazelnuts, toasted, peeled, and coarsely chopped (see How To Toast and Skin Nuts)

1. Preheat the oven to 300°F. Grease 2 large baking sheets.

2. In a large bowl, with an electric mixer at medium speed, beat the egg whites and salt until foamy. Increase the speed to high and gradually add the sugar. Beat until soft peaks form when the beaters are lifted.

3. On low speed, mix in the cocoa. Stir in the hazelnuts.

4. Scrape the mixture into a large heavy saucepan. Cook over medium heat, stirring constantly with a wooden spoon, until the mixture is shiny and smooth, about 5 minutes. Be careful that it does not scorch.

5. Immediately drop the hot batter by tablespoonfuls onto the prepared baking sheets. Bake 30 minutes or until firm and slightly cracked on the surface.

6. While the cookies are still hot, transfer them to a rack to cool, using a thin-blade metal spatula. Store in an airtight container up to 2 weeks.

Double-Chocolate Nut Biscotti

Biscotti al Cioccolato

Makes 4 dozen

These rich biscotti have chocolate in the dough, both melted and in chunks. I have never seen them in Italy, but they are similar to what I have tasted in coffee bars here.

2½ cups all-purpose flour

2 teaspoons baking powder

½ teaspoon salt

3 large eggs, at room temperature

1 cup sugar

1 teaspoon pure vanilla extract

6 ounces bittersweet chocolate, melted and cooled

6 tablespoons (½ stick plus 2 tablespoons) unsalted butter, melted and cooled

1 cup walnuts, coarsely chopped

1 cup chocolate chips

1. Place a rack in the center of the oven. Preheat the oven to 300°F. Grease and flour 2 large baking sheets.

2. In a large bowl, sift together the flour, baking powder, and salt.

3. In a large bowl, with an electric mixer at medium speed, beat the eggs, sugar, and vanilla until foamy and light, about 2 minutes. Stir in the chocolate and butter until blended. Add the flour mixture and stir until smooth, about 1 minute more. Stir in the nuts and chocolate chips.

4. Divide the dough in half. With moistened hands, shape each piece into a 12 × 3–inch log on the prepared baking sheet. Bake for 35 minutes or until the logs are firm when pressed in the center. Remove the pan from the oven, but do not turn off the heat. Let cool 10 minutes.

5. Slide the logs onto a cutting board. Cut the logs into $1/2$-inch-thick slices. Lay the slices on the baking sheet. Bake for 10 minutes or until the cookies are lightly toasted.

6. Have ready 2 large cooling racks. Transfer the baking sheets to the racks. Let the cookies cool 5 minutes on the baking sheets,

then transfer them to the racks to cool completely. Store in an airtight container up to 2 weeks.

Chocolate Kisses

Baci di Cioccolato

Makes 3 dozen

Chocolate and vanilla "kisses" are a favorite in Verona, home of Romeo and Juliet, where they are made in a variety of combinations.

1⅔ cups all-purpose flour

⅓ cup unsweetened Dutch-process cocoa powder, sifted

¼ teaspoon salt

1 cup (2 sticks) unsalted butter, at room temperature

½ cup confectioner's sugar

1 teaspoon pure vanilla extract

½ cup finely chopped toasted almonds (see How To Toast and Skin Nuts)

Filling

2 ounces semisweet or bittersweet chocolate, chopped

2 tablespoons unsalted butter

⅓ cup almonds, toasted and finely chopped

1. In a large bowl, sift together the flour, cocoa, and salt.

2. In a large bowl, with an electric mixer at medium speed, beat the butter and sugar until light and fluffy, about 2 minutes. Beat in the vanilla. Stir in the dry ingredients and the almonds until blended, about 1 minute more. Cover with plastic and chill in the refrigerator 1 hour up to overnight.

3. Preheat the oven to 350°F. Have ready 2 ungreased baking sheets. Roll teaspoonfuls of the dough into ¾-inch balls. Place the balls 1 inch apart on the baking sheets. With your fingers, press the balls to flatten them slightly. Bake the cookies until firm but not browned, 10 to 12 minutes. Have ready 2 large cooling racks.

4. Transfer the baking sheets to the racks. Let the cookies cool 5 minutes on the baking sheets, then transfer them to the racks to cool completely.

5. Bring about 2 inches of water to a simmer in the bottom half of a double boiler or a small saucepan. Place the chocolate and the butter in the top half of the double boiler or in a small heatproof bowl that fits comfortably over the saucepan. Place the bowl over the simmering water. Let stand uncovered until the chocolate is softened. Stir until smooth. Stir in the almonds.

6. Spread a small amount of the filling mixture on the bottom of one cookie. Place a second cookie bottom-side down on the filling and press together lightly. Place the cookies on a wire rack until the filling is set. Repeat with the remaining cookies and filling. Store in an airtight container in the refrigerator up to 1 week.

No-Bake Chocolate "Salame"

Salame del Cioccolato

Makes 32 cookies

Crunchy chocolate nut slices that require no baking are a specialty of Piedmont. Other cookies can be substituted for the amaretti, if you prefer, such as vanilla or chocolate wafers, graham crackers, or shortbread. These are best made a few days ahead, to allow the flavors to blend. If you prefer not use the liqueur, substitute a spoonful of orange juice.

18 amaretti cookies

1/3 cup sugar

1/3 cup unsweetened cocoa powder

1/2 cup (1 stick) unsalted butter, softened

1 tablespoon grappa or rum

1/3 cup chopped walnuts

1. Place the cookies in a plastic bag. Crush the cookies with a rolling pin or heavy object. There should be about 3/4 cup of crumbs.

2. Place the crumbs in a large bowl. With a wooden spoon, stir in the sugar and cocoa. Add the butter and grappa. Stir until the dry ingredients are moistened and blended. Stir in the walnuts.

3. Place a 14-inch sheet of plastic wrap on a flat surface. Pour the dough mixture onto the plastic wrap. Shape the dough into an 8 × $2^1/_2$–inch log. Roll the log in the plastic wrap, folding the ends over to enclose it completely. Refrigerate the log at least 24 hours and up to 3 days.

4. Cut the log into $1/_4$-inch-thick slices. Serve chilled. Store the cookies in an airtight plastic container in the refrigerator up to 2 weeks.

Prato Biscuits

Biscotti di Prato

Makes about 4½ dozen

In the town of Prato in Tuscany, these are the classic biscotti to dip in vin santo, the great dessert wine of the region. Eaten plain, they are rather dry, so do provide a beverage for dunking them.

2½ cups all-purpose flour

1½ teaspoons baking powder

1 teaspoon salt

4 large eggs

¾ cup sugar

1 teaspoon grated lemon zest

1 teaspoon grated orange zest

1 teaspoon pure vanilla extract

1 cup toasted almonds (see How To Toast and Skin Nuts)

1. Place a rack in the center of the oven. Preheat the oven to 325°F. Grease and flour a large baking sheet.

2. In a medium bowl, sift together the flour, baking powder, and salt.

3. In a large bowl with an electric mixer, beat the eggs and sugar on medium speed until light and foamy, about 3 minutes. Beat in the lemon and orange zests and vanilla. On low speed, stir in the dry ingredients, then stir in the almonds.

4. Lightly dampen your hands. Shape the dough into two 14 × 2-inch logs. Place the logs on the prepared baking sheet several inches apart. Bake for 30 minutes or until firm and golden.

5. Remove the baking sheet from the oven and reduce the oven heat to 300°F. Let the logs cool on the baking sheet for 20 minutes.

6. Slide the logs onto a cutting board. With a large heavy chef's knife, cut the logs on the diagonal into $1/2$-inch-thick slices. Lay the slices on the baking sheet. Bake 20 minutes or until lightly golden.

7. Transfer the cookies to wire racks to cool. Store in an airtight container.

Umbrian Fruit and Nut Biscotti

Tozzetti

Makes 80

Made without fat, these cookies keep a long time in an airtight container. The flavor actually improves, so plan to make them several days before serving them.

3 cups all-purpose flour

½ cup cornstarch

2 teaspoons baking powder

3 large eggs

3 egg yolks

2 tablespoons Marsala, vin santo, or sherry

1 cup sugar

1 cup raisins

1 cup almonds

¼ cup chopped candied orange peel

¼ cup chopped candied citron

1 teaspoon anise seeds

1. Preheat the oven to 350°F. Grease 2 large baking sheets.

2. In a medium bowl, sift together the flour, cornstarch, and baking powder.

3. In a large bowl with an electric mixer, beat together the eggs, yolks, and Marsala. Add the sugar and beat until well blended, about 3 minutes. Stir in the dry ingredients, the raisins, almonds, peel, citron and anise seeds until blended. The dough will be stiff. If necessary, turn the dough out onto a countertop and knead it until blended.

4. Divide the dough into quarters. Dampen your hands with cool water and shape each quarter into a 10-inch log. Place the logs 2 inches apart on the prepared baking sheets.

5. Bake the logs 20 minutes or until they feel firm when pressed in the center and are golden brown around the edges. Remove the logs from the oven but leave the oven on. Let the logs cool 5 minutes on the baking sheets.

6. Slide the logs onto a cutting board. With a large chef's knife, cut them into $1/2$-inch-thick slices. Place the slices on the baking sheets and bake 10 minutes or until lightly toasted.

7. Have ready 2 large cooling racks. Transfer the cookies to the racks. Let cool completely. Store in an airtight container up to 2 weeks.

Butter Rings

Bussolai

Makes 36

These Venetian cookies are simple to make and a pleasure to have around the house for a midday snack or whenever guests stop in.

1 cup sugar

½ cup (1 stick) unsalted butter, at room temperature

3 large egg yolks

1 teaspoon grated lemon zest

1 teaspoon grated orange zest

1 teaspoon pure vanilla extract

2 cups all-purpose flour

½ teaspoon salt

1 egg white, beaten until foamy

1. Set aside $1/3$ cup of the sugar.

2. In the large bowl of an electric mixer, beat the butter with the remaining ⅔ cup of sugar at medium speed until light and fluffy, about 2 minutes. Beat in the egg yolks one at a time. Add the lemon and orange zests and vanilla extract and beat, scraping the sides of the bowl, until smooth, about 2 minutes more.

3. Stir in the flour and salt until well blended. Shape the dough into a ball. Wrap in plastic wrap and refrigerate 1 hour up to overnight.

4. Preheat the oven to 325°F. Grease 2 large baking sheets. Cut the dough into 6 pieces. Divide each piece again into 6 pieces. Roll each piece into a 4-inch rope, shape into a ring, and pinch the ends together to seal. Place the rings 1 inch apart on the prepared baking sheets. Brush lightly with the egg white and sprinkle with the reserved ⅓ cup of sugar.

5. Bake 15 minutes or until lightly browned. Have ready 2 wire cooling racks.

6. Transfer the baking sheets to the racks. Let the cookies cool 5 minutes on the baking sheets, then transfer them to the wire racks to cool completely. Store in an airtight container up to 2 weeks.

Lemon Knots

Tarralucci

Makes 40

Every Italian bakery in Brooklyn, New York, made these refreshing Sicilian lemon cookies when I was growing up. I like to serve them with iced tea.

If the weather is hot and humid, the icing may refuse to firm up at room temperature. In that case, store the cookies in the refrigerator.

4 cups all-purpose flour

4 teaspoons baking powder

1 cup sugar

½ cup solid vegetable shortening

3 large eggs

½ cup milk

2 tablespoons lemon juice

2 teaspoons grated lemon zest

Icing

1½ cups confectioner's sugar

1 tablespoon freshly squeezed lemon juice

2 teaspoons grated lemon zest

Milk

1. Sift together the flour and baking powder onto a piece of wax paper.

2. In a large bowl, with an electric mixer at medium speed, beat the sugar and shortening until light and fluffy, about 2 minutes. Beat in the eggs one at a time until well blended. Stir in the milk, lemon juice, and zest. Scrape the sides of the bowl. Stir in the dry ingredients until smooth, about 2 minutes. Cover with plastic wrap and refrigerate at least 1 hour.

3. Preheat the oven to 350°F. Have ready 2 large baking sheets. Pinch off a piece of dough the size of a golf ball. Lightly roll the dough into a 6-inch rope. Tie the rope into a knot. Place the knot on an ungreased baking sheet. Continue making the knots and placing them about 1 inch apart on the sheets.

4. Bake the cookies 12 minutes or until firm when pressed on top but not browned. Have ready 2 wire cooling racks.

5. Transfer the baking sheets to the racks. Let the cookies cool 5 minutes on the baking sheets, then transfer them to the wire racks to cool completely.

6. Combine the confectioner's sugar, lemon juice, and zest in a large bowl. Add milk 1 teaspoon at a time and stir until the mixture forms a thin icing with the consistency of heavy cream.

7. Dip the tops of the cookies in the icing. Place them on a rack until the icing is hardened. Store in airtight containers up to 3 days.

Spice Cookies

Bicciolani

Makes 75

In caffès in Turin you can order barbajada, a combination of half coffee and half hot chocolate. It would be perfect with these thin, buttery spice cookies.

1 cup (2 sticks) unsalted butter, at room temperature

1 cup sugar

1 egg yolk

2 cups all-purpose flour

½ teaspoon salt

1 teaspoon ground cinnamon

⅛ teaspoon freshly grated nutmeg

⅛ teaspoon ground cloves

1. Preheat the oven to 350°F. Grease a 15 × 10 × 1– inch jelly roll pan.

2. In a bowl, stir together the flour, salt, and spices.

3. In a large electric mixer bowl, beat the butter, sugar, and egg yolk on medium speed until light and fluffy, about 2 minutes. Reduce the speed to low and stir in the dry ingredients until thoroughly blended, about 2 minutes more.

4. Crumble the dough into the prepared pan. With your hands, firmly press the dough out into an even layer. With the back of a fork, make shallow ridges in the top of the dough.

5. Bake 25 to 30 minutes or until lightly browned. Transfer the pan to a wire cooling rack. Cool 10 minutes. Then cut the dough into 2 × 1–inch cookies.

6. Cool completely in the pan. Store at room temperature in an airtight container up to 2 weeks.

Wafer Cookies

Pizzelle

Makes about 2 dozen

Many families in central and southern Italy are proud of their pizzelle irons, beautifully crafted forms traditionally used to make these pretty wafers. Some irons are embossed with the original owner's initials, while others have silhouettes such as a couple toasting each other with a glass of wine. They were once a typical wedding gift.

Though charming, these old fashioned irons are heavy and unwieldy on today's stoves. An electric pizzelle press, similar to a waffle iron, does an efficient and quick job of turning out these cookies.

When they are freshly made, pizzelle are pliable and can be molded into cone, tube, or cup shapes. They can be filled with whipped cream, ice cream, cannoli cream, or fruit. They cool and crisp in no time, so you must work quickly and carefully to shape them. Of course, they are good flat as well.

1¾ cups unbleached all-purpose flour

1 teaspoon baking powder

Pinch of salt

3 large eggs

⅔ cup sugar

1 tablespoon pure vanilla extract

1 stick (½ cup) unsalted butter, melted and cooled

1. Preheat the pizzelle maker according to the manufacturer's directions. In a bowl, stir together the flour, baking powder, and salt.

2. In a large bowl, beat the eggs, sugar, and vanilla with an electric mixer on medium speed until thick and light, about 4 minutes. Beat in the butter. Stir in the dry ingredients until just blended, about 1 minute.

3. Place about 1 tablespoon of the batter in the center of each pizzelle mold. (The exact amount will depend on the design of the mold.) Close the cover and bake until lightly golden. This will depend on the maker and how long the mold has been heating. Check it carefully after 30 seconds.

4. When the pizzelle are golden, slide them off the molds with a wooden or plastic spatula. Let cool flat on a wire rack. Or, to

make cookie cups, bend each pizzelle into the curve of a wide coffee or dessert cup. To make cannoli shells, shape them around cannoli tubes or a wooden dowel.

5. When the pizzelle are cool and crisp, store them in an airtight container until ready to use. These last for several weeks.

Variation: *Anise*: Substitute 1 tablespoon anise extract and 1 tablespoon anise seeds for the vanilla. *Orange or Lemon*: Add 1 tablespoon grated fresh orange or lemon zest to the egg mixture. *Rum or Almond*: Stir in 1 tablespoon rum or almond extract instead of the vanilla. *Nut*: Stir in $1/4$ cup of nuts ground to a very fine powder along with the flour.

Sweet Ravioli

Ravioli Dolci

Makes 2 dozen

Jam fills these crisp dessert ravioli. Any flavor will do, as long as it has a thick consistency so that it will stay in place and not ooze out of the dough as it bakes. This was a favorite recipe of my father, who perfected it from his memories of the cookies his mother used to make.

1¾ cup all-purpose flour

½ cup potato or corn starch

½ teaspoon salt

½ cup (1 stick) unsalted butter, at room temperature

½ cup sugar

1 large egg

2 tablespoons rum or brandy

1 teaspoon grated lemon zest

1 teaspoon pure vanilla extract

1 cup thick sour cherry, raspberry, or apricot jam

1. In a large bowl, sift together the flour, starch, and salt.

2. In a large bowl with an electric mixer, beat the butter with the sugar until light and fluffy, about 2 minutes. Beat in the egg, rum, zest, and vanilla. On low speed, stir in the dry ingredients.

3. Divide the dough in half. Shape each half into a disk. Wrap each separately in plastic and refrigerate 1 hour up to overnight.

4. Preheat the oven to 350°F. Grease 2 large baking sheets.

5. Roll out the dough to a $1/8$-inch thickness. With a fluted pastry or pasta cutter, cut the dough into 2-inch squares. Arrange the squares about 1 inch apart on the prepared baking sheets. Place $1/2$ teaspoon of the jam in the center of each square. (Do not use more jam, or the filling will leak out as it bakes.)

6. Roll out the remaining dough to a $1/8$-inch thickness. Cut the dough into 2-inch squares.

7. Cover the jam with the dough squares. Press the edges all around with a fork to seal in the filling.

8. Bake 16 to 18 minutes, or until lightly browned. Have ready 2 wire cooling racks.

9. Transfer the baking sheets to the racks. Let the cookies cool 5 minutes on the baking sheets, then transfer them to the wire racks to cool completely. Sprinkle with confectioner's sugar. Store in an airtight container up to 1 week.

"Ugly-but-Good" Cookies

Brutti ma Buoni

Makes 2 dozen

"Ugly but good" is the meaning of the name of these Piedmontese cookies. The name is only half-true: The cookies are not ugly, but they are good. The technique for making these is unusual. The cookie batter is cooked in a saucepan before it is baked.

3 large egg whites, at room temperature

Pinch of salt

1½ cups sugar

1 cup unsweetened cocoa powder

1¼ cups hazelnuts, toasted, peeled, and coarsely chopped (see How To Toast and Skin Nuts)

1. Preheat the oven to 300°F. Grease 2 large baking sheets.

2. In a large bowl, with an electric mixer at medium speed, beat the egg whites and salt until foamy. Increase the speed to high and gradually add the sugar. Beat until soft peaks form when the beaters are lifted.

3. On low speed, mix in the cocoa. Stir in the hazelnuts.

4. Scrape the mixture into a large heavy saucepan. Cook over medium heat, stirring constantly with a wooden spoon, until the mixture is shiny and smooth, about 5 minutes. Be careful that it does not scorch.

5. Immediately drop the hot batter by tablespoonfuls onto the prepared baking sheets. Bake 30 minutes or until firm and slightly cracked on the surface.

6. While the cookies are still hot, transfer them to a rack to cool, using a thin-blade metal spatula. Store in an airtight container up to 2 weeks.

Jam Spots

Biscotti di Marmellata

Makes 40

Chocolate, nuts, and jam are a winning combination in these tasty cookies. They are always a hit on Christmas cookie trays.

¾ cup (1½ sticks) unsalted butter, at room temperature

½ cup sugar

½ teaspoon salt

3 ounces bittersweet chocolate, melted and cooled

2 cups all-purpose flour

¾ cup finely chopped almonds

½ cup thick seedless raspberry jam

1. Preheat the oven to 350°F. Grease 2 large baking sheets.

2. In a large bowl, with an electric mixer on medium speed, beat the butter, sugar, and salt until light and fluffy, about 2 minutes.

Add the melted chocolate and beat until well blended, scraping the sides of the bowl. Stir in the flour until smooth.

3. Place the nuts in a shallow bowl. Shape the dough into 1-inch balls. Roll the balls in the nuts, pressing lightly so they will adhere. Place the balls about $1^1/_2$ inches apart on the prepared baking sheets.

4. With the handle end of a wooden spoon, poke a deep hole in each ball of dough, molding the dough around the handle to maintain the round shape. Place about $^1/_4$ teaspoon jam in each cookie. (Do not add more jam, as it may melt and leak out when the cookies bake.)

5. Bake the cookies 18 to 20 minutes, or until the jam is bubbling and the cookies are lightly browned. Have ready 2 wire cooling racks.

6. Transfer the baking sheets to the racks. Let the cookies cool 5 minutes on the baking sheets, then transfer them to the wire racks to cool completely. Store in an airtight container up to 2 weeks.

Double-Chocolate Nut Biscotti

Biscotti al Cioccolato

Makes 4 dozen

These rich biscotti have chocolate in the dough, both melted and in chunks. I have never seen them in Italy, but they are similar to what I have tasted in coffee bars here.

2½ cups all-purpose flour

2 teaspoons baking powder

½ teaspoon salt

3 large eggs, at room temperature

1 cup sugar

1 teaspoon pure vanilla extract

6 ounces bittersweet chocolate, melted and cooled

6 tablespoons (½ stick plus 2 tablespoons) unsalted butter, melted and cooled

1 cup walnuts, coarsely chopped

1 cup chocolate chips

1. Place a rack in the center of the oven. Preheat the oven to 300°F. Grease and flour 2 large baking sheets.

2. In a large bowl, sift together the flour, baking powder, and salt.

3. In a large bowl, with an electric mixer at medium speed, beat the eggs, sugar, and vanilla until foamy and light, about 2 minutes. Stir in the chocolate and butter until blended. Add the flour mixture and stir until smooth, about 1 minute more. Stir in the nuts and chocolate chips.

4. Divide the dough in half. With moistened hands, shape each piece into a 12 × 3-inch log on the prepared baking sheet. Bake for 35 minutes or until the logs are firm when pressed in the center. Remove the pan from the oven, but do not turn off the heat. Let cool 10 minutes.

5. Slide the logs onto a cutting board. Cut the logs into $1/2$-inch-thick slices. Lay the slices on the baking sheet. Bake for 10 minutes or until the cookies are lightly toasted.

6. Have ready 2 large cooling racks. Transfer the baking sheets to the racks. Let the cookies cool 5 minutes on the baking sheets,

then transfer them to the racks to cool completely. Store in an airtight container up to 2 weeks.

Chocolate Kisses

Baci di Cioccolato

Makes 3 dozen

Chocolate and vanilla "kisses" are a favorite in Verona, home of Romeo and Juliet, where they are made in a variety of combinations.

1⅔ cups all-purpose flour

⅓ cup unsweetened Dutch-process cocoa powder, sifted

¼ teaspoon salt

1 cup (2 sticks) unsalted butter, at room temperature

½ cup confectioner's sugar

1 teaspoon pure vanilla extract

½ cup finely chopped toasted almonds (see How To Toast and Skin Nuts)

Filling

2 ounces semisweet or bittersweet chocolate, chopped

2 tablespoons unsalted butter

⅓ cup almonds, toasted and finely chopped

1. In a large bowl, sift together the flour, cocoa, and salt.

2. In a large bowl, with an electric mixer at medium speed, beat the butter and sugar until light and fluffy, about 2 minutes. Beat in the vanilla. Stir in the dry ingredients and the almonds until blended, about 1 minute more. Cover with plastic and chill in the refrigerator 1 hour up to overnight.

3. Preheat the oven to 350°F. Have ready 2 ungreased baking sheets. Roll teaspoonfuls of the dough into ¾-inch balls. Place the balls 1 inch apart on the baking sheets. With your fingers, press the balls to flatten them slightly. Bake the cookies until firm but not browned, 10 to 12 minutes. Have ready 2 large cooling racks.

4. Transfer the baking sheets to the racks. Let the cookies cool 5 minutes on the baking sheets, then transfer them to the racks to cool completely.

5. Bring about 2 inches of water to a simmer in the bottom half of a double boiler or a small saucepan. Place the chocolate and the butter in the top half of the double boiler or in a small heatproof bowl that fits comfortably over the saucepan. Place the bowl

over the simmering water. Let stand uncovered until the chocolate is softened. Stir until smooth. Stir in the almonds.

6. Spread a small amount of the filling mixture on the bottom of one cookie. Place a second cookie bottom-side down on the filling and press together lightly. Place the cookies on a wire rack until the filling is set. Repeat with the remaining cookies and filling. Store in an airtight container in the refrigerator up to 1 week.

No-Bake Chocolate "Salame"

Salame del Cioccolato

Makes 32 cookies

Crunchy chocolate nut slices that require no baking are a specialty of Piedmont. Other cookies can be substituted for the amaretti, if you prefer, such as vanilla or chocolate wafers, graham crackers, or shortbread. These are best made a few days ahead, to allow the flavors to blend. If you prefer not use the liqueur, substitute a spoonful of orange juice.

18 amaretti cookies

⅓ cup sugar

⅓ cup unsweetened cocoa powder

½ cup (1 stick) unsalted butter, softened

1 tablespoon grappa or rum

⅓ cup chopped walnuts

1. Place the cookies in a plastic bag. Crush the cookies with a rolling pin or heavy object. There should be about ¾ cup of crumbs.

2. Place the crumbs in a large bowl. With a wooden spoon, stir in the sugar and cocoa. Add the butter and grappa. Stir until the dry ingredients are moistened and blended. Stir in the walnuts.

3. Place a 14-inch sheet of plastic wrap on a flat surface. Pour the dough mixture onto the plastic wrap. Shape the dough into an 8 × 2$\frac{1}{2}$–inch log. Roll the log in the plastic wrap, folding the ends over to enclose it completely. Refrigerate the log at least 24 hours and up to 3 days.

4. Cut the log into $\frac{1}{4}$-inch-thick slices. Serve chilled. Store the cookies in an airtight plastic container in the refrigerator up to 2 weeks.

Prato Biscuits

Biscotti di Prato

Makes about 4½ dozen

In the town of Prato in Tuscany, these are the classic biscotti to dip in vin santo, the great dessert wine of the region. Eaten plain, they are rather dry, so do provide a beverage for dunking them.

2½ cups all-purpose flour

1½ teaspoons baking powder

1 teaspoon salt

4 large eggs

¾ cup sugar

1 teaspoon grated lemon zest

1 teaspoon grated orange zest

1 teaspoon pure vanilla extract

1 cup toasted almonds (see How To Toast and Skin Nuts)

1. Place a rack in the center of the oven. Preheat the oven to 325°F. Grease and flour a large baking sheet.

2. In a medium bowl, sift together the flour, baking powder, and salt.

3. In a large bowl with an electric mixer, beat the eggs and sugar on medium speed until light and foamy, about 3 minutes. Beat in the lemon and orange zests and vanilla. On low speed, stir in the dry ingredients, then stir in the almonds.

4. Lightly dampen your hands. Shape the dough into two 14 × 2-inch logs. Place the logs on the prepared baking sheet several inches apart. Bake for 30 minutes or until firm and golden.

5. Remove the baking sheet from the oven and reduce the oven heat to 300°F. Let the logs cool on the baking sheet for 20 minutes.

6. Slide the logs onto a cutting board. With a large heavy chef's knife, cut the logs on the diagonal into $1/2$-inch-thick slices. Lay the slices on the baking sheet. Bake 20 minutes or until lightly golden.

7. Transfer the cookies to wire racks to cool. Store in an airtight container.

Umbrian Fruit and Nut Biscotti

Tozzetti

Makes 80

Made without fat, these cookies keep a long time in an airtight container. The flavor actually improves, so plan to make them several days before serving them.

3 cups all-purpose flour

½ cup cornstarch

2 teaspoons baking powder

3 large eggs

3 egg yolks

2 tablespoons Marsala, vin santo, or sherry

1 cup sugar

1 cup raisins

1 cup almonds

¼ cup chopped candied orange peel

¼ cup chopped candied citron

1 teaspoon anise seeds

1. Preheat the oven to 350°F. Grease 2 large baking sheets.

2. In a medium bowl, sift together the flour, cornstarch, and baking powder.

3. In a large bowl with an electric mixer, beat together the eggs, yolks, and Marsala. Add the sugar and beat until well blended, about 3 minutes. Stir in the dry ingredients, the raisins, almonds, peel, citron and anise seeds until blended. The dough will be stiff. If necessary, turn the dough out onto a countertop and knead it until blended.

4. Divide the dough into quarters. Dampen your hands with cool water and shape each quarter into a 10-inch log. Place the logs 2 inches apart on the prepared baking sheets.

5. Bake the logs 20 minutes or until they feel firm when pressed in the center and are golden brown around the edges. Remove the logs from the oven but leave the oven on. Let the logs cool 5 minutes on the baking sheets.

6. Slide the logs onto a cutting board. With a large chef's knife, cut them into $1/2$-inch-thick slices. Place the slices on the baking sheets and bake 10 minutes or until lightly toasted.

7. Have ready 2 large cooling racks. Transfer the cookies to the racks. Let cool completely. Store in an airtight container up to 2 weeks.

Lemon Nut Biscotti

Biscotti al Limone

Makes 48

Lemon and almonds flavor these biscotti.

1½ cups all-purpose flour

1 teaspoon baking powder

¼ teaspoon salt

½ cup (1 stick) unsalted butter, at room temperature

½ cup sugar

2 large eggs, at room temperature

2 teaspoons freshly grated lemon zest

1 cup toasted almonds, coarsely chopped

1. Place a rack in the center of the oven. Preheat the oven to 350°F. Grease and flour a large baking sheet.

2. In a bowl, sift together the flour, baking powder, and salt.

3. In a large bowl with an electric mixer, beat the butter and sugar until light and fluffy, about 2 minutes. Beat in the eggs one at a time. Add the lemon zest, scraping the inside of the bowl with a rubber spatula. Gradually stir in the flour mixture and the nuts until blended.

4. Divide the dough in half. With moistened hands, shape each piece into a 12 × 2–inch log on the prepared baking sheet. Bake for 20 minutes or until the logs are lightly browned and firm when pressed in the center. Remove the pan from the oven, but do not turn off the heat. Let the logs cool 10 minutes on the baking sheet.

5. Slide the logs onto a cutting board. Cut the logs into $1/2$-inch-thick slices. Place the slices on the baking sheet. Bake for 10 minutes or until the cookies are lightly toasted.

6. Have ready 2 large cooling racks. Transfer the cookies to the racks. Let cool completely. Store in an airtight container up to 2 weeks.

Walnut Biscotti

Biscotti di Noce

Makes about 80

Olive oil can be used for baking in a wide range of recipes. Use a mild-flavored extra-virgin olive oil. It complements many types of nuts and citrus fruits. Here is a biscotti recipe I developed for an article in the Washington Post about baking with olive oil.

2 cups all-purpose flour

1 teaspoon baking powder

1 teaspoon salt

2 large eggs, at room temperature

⅔ cup sugar

½ cup extra-virgin olive oil

½ teaspoon grated lemon zest

2 cups toasted walnuts (see How To Toast and Skin Nuts)

1. Preheat the oven to 325°F. Grease 2 large baking sheets.

2. In a large bowl, combine the flour, baking powder, and salt.

3. In another large bowl, whisk the eggs, sugar, oil, and lemon zest until well blended. With a wooden spoon, stir in the dry ingredients just until blended. Stir in the walnuts.

4. Divide the dough into four pieces. Shape the pieces into 12 × 1 1/2–inch logs, placing them several inches apart on the prepared baking sheets. Bake for 20 to 25 minutes or until lightly browned. Remove from the oven, but do not turn it off. Let the cookies cool on the baking sheets 10 minutes.

5. Slide the logs onto a cutting board. With a large heavy knife, cut the logs diagonally into 1/2-inch slices. Lay the slices on the baking sheets and return the sheets to the oven. Bake 10 minutes or until toasted and golden.

6. Have ready 2 large cooling racks. Transfer the cookies to the racks. Let cool completely. Store in an airtight container up to 2 weeks.

Almond Macaroons

Amaretti

Makes 3 dozen

In southern Italy, these are made by grinding up both sweet and bitter almonds. Bitter almonds, which come from a particular variety of almond tree, are not sold in the United States. They have a flavor component similar to cyanide, a lethal poison, so they are not approved for commercial use. The closest we can come to the correct flavor is commercial almond paste and a little almond extract. Do not confuse almond paste with marzipan, which is similar, but has a higher sugar content. Buy the almond paste sold in cans for best flavor. If you can't find it, ask at your local bakery to see if they will sell you some.

These cookies stick, so I bake them on nonstick baking mats known as Silpat. The mats never need greasing, are easy to clean, and reusable. You can find them at good kitchen supply stores. If you don't have the mats, the baking pans can be lined with parchment paper or aluminum foil.

1 (8-ounce) can almond paste, crumbled

1 cup sugar

2 large egg whites, at room temperature

¼ teaspoon almond extract

36 candied cherries or whole almonds

1. Preheat the oven to 350°F. Line 2 large baking sheets with parchment paper or aluminum foil.

2. Crumble the almond paste into a large bowl. With an electric mixer on low speed, beat in the sugar until blended. Add the egg whites and almond extract. Increase the speed to medium and beat until very smooth, about 3 minutes.

3. Scoop up 1 tablespoon of the batter and lightly roll it into a ball. Dampen your fingertips with cool water if necessary to prevent sticking. Place the balls about one inch apart on the prepared baking sheet. Press a cherry or almond into the top of the dough.

4. Bake 18 to 20 minutes or until the cookies are lightly browned. Let cool briefly on the baking sheet.

5. With a thin metal spatula, transfer the cookies to wire racks to cool completely. Store the cookies in airtight containers. (If you want to keep these cookies for more than a day or two, freeze

them to maintain their soft texture. They can be eaten directly from the freezer.)

Pine Nut Macaroons

Biscotti di Pinoli

Makes 40

I have made many variations of these cookies over the years. This version is my favorite because it is made with both almond paste and ground almonds for both flavor and texture and has the added rich flavor of toasted pine nuts (pignoli).

1 (8-ounce) can almond paste

⅓ cup finely ground blanched almonds

2 large egg whites

1 cup confectioner's sugar, plus more for decorating

2 cups pine nuts or slivered almonds

1. Place a rack in the center of the oven. Preheat the oven to 350°F. Grease a large baking sheet.

2. In a large bowl, crumble the almond paste. With an electric mixer on medium speed, beat in the almonds, egg whites, and 1 cup of confectioner's sugar until smooth.

3. Scoop up a tablespoon of the batter. Roll the batter in the pine nuts, covering it completely and forming a ball. Place the ball on the prepared baking sheet. Repeat with the remaining ingredients, placing the balls about 1 inch apart.

4. Bake 18 to 20 minutes or until lightly browned. Place the baking sheet on a cooling rack. Let the cookies cool 2 minutes on the baking sheet.

5. Transfer the cookies to racks to cool completely. Dust with confectioner's sugar. Store in an airtight container in the refrigerator up to 1 week.

Hazelnut Bars

Nocciolate

Makes 6 dozen

These tender, crumbly bars are packed with nuts. They barely hold together and melt in the mouth. Serve them with chocolate ice cream.

2 ⅓ cups all-purpose flour

1½ cups peeled, toasted hazelnuts, finely chopped (see How To Toast and Skin Nuts)

1½ cups sugar

½ teaspoon salt

1 cup (2 sticks) unsalted butter, melted and cooled

1 large egg plus 1 egg yolk, beaten

1. Place a rack in the center of the oven. Preheat the oven to 350°F. Grease a 15 × 10 × 1–inch jelly roll pan.

2. In a large bowl with a wooden spoon, stir together the flour, nuts, sugar, and salt. Add the butter and stir until evenly moistened. Add the eggs. Stir until well blended and the mixture holds together.

3. Pour the mixture into the prepared pan. Firmly pat it out into an even layer.

4. Bake 30 minutes or until golden brown. While still hot, cut into 2 × 1-inch rectangles.

5. Let cool 10 minutes in the pan. Transfer the cookies to large racks to cool completely.

Walnut Butter Cookies

Biscotti di Noce

Makes 5 dozen

Nutty and buttery, these crescent-shaped cookies from Piedmont are perfect for Christmas. Though they are often made with hazelnuts, I like to use walnuts. Almonds can also be substituted.

These cookies can be made entirely in the food processor. If you don't have one, grind the nuts and sugar in a blender or nut grinder, then stir in the remaining ingredients by hand.

1 cup walnut pieces

⅓ cup sugar plus 1 cup more for rolling the cookies

2 cups all-purpose flour

1 cup (2 sticks) unsalted butter, at room temperature

1. Preheat oven to 350°F. Grease and flour 2 large baking sheets.

2. In a food processor, combine the walnuts and sugar. Process until the nuts are finely chopped. Add the flour and process until blended.

3. Add the butter a little at a time and pulse to blend. Remove the dough from the container and squeeze it together with your hands.

4. Pour the remaining 1 cup of sugar into a shallow bowl. Pinch off a piece of dough the size of a walnut and form it into a ball. Shape the ball into a crescent, tapering the ends. Gently roll the crescent in sugar. Place the crescent on a prepared baking sheet. Repeat with the remaining dough and sugar, placing each cookie about 1 inch apart.

5. Bake 15 minutes or until lightly browned. Place the baking sheets on wire racks to cool 5 minutes.

6. Transfer the cookies to the racks to cool completely. Store in an airtight container up to 2 weeks.

Rainbow Cookies

Biscotti Tricolori

Makes about 4 dozen

Though I have never seen them in Italy, these "rainbow," or tricolored, cookies with a chocolate glaze are a favorite at Italian and other bakeries in the United States. Unfortunately, they are often colored garishly and can be dry and tasteless.

Try this recipe and you will see how good these cookies can be. They are a bit fussy to make, but the results are very pretty and delicious. If you prefer not to use food coloring, the cookies will still be attractive. For convenience, it is best to have three identical baking pans. But you can still make the cookies with only one pan if you bake one batch of dough at a time. The finished cookies keep well in the refrigerator.

8 ounces almond paste

1½ cups (3 sticks) unsalted butter

1 cup sugar

4 large eggs, separated

¼ teaspoon salt

2 cups unbleached all-purpose flour

10 drops red food coloring, or to taste (optional)

10 drops green food coloring, or to taste (optional)

½ cup apricot preserves

½ cup seedless raspberry jam

1 (6-ounce) package semisweet chocolate chips

1. Preheat the oven to 350°F. Grease three 13 × 9 × 2–inch identical baking pans. Line the pans with wax paper and grease the paper.

2. Crumble the almond paste into a large mixer bowl. Add the butter, $1/2$ cup of the sugar, the egg yolks, and salt. Beat until light and fluffy. Stir in the flour just until blended.

3. In another large bowl, with clean beaters, beat the egg whites on medium speed until foamy. Gradually beat in the remaining sugar. Increase the speed to high. Continue beating until the egg whites form soft peaks when the beaters are lifted.

4. With a rubber spatula, fold $1/3$ of the whites into the yolk mixture to lighten it. Gradually fold in the remaining whites.

5. Scoop $1/3$ of the batter into one bowl, and another $1/3$ into another bowl. If using the food coloring, fold the red into one bowl and the green into the other.

6. Spread each bowl of batter into a separate prepared pan, smoothing it out evenly with a spatula. Bake the layers 10 to 12 minutes, until the cake is just set and very lightly colored around the edges. Let cool in the pan for 5 minutes, then lift the layers onto cooling racks, leaving the wax paper attached. Let cool completely.

7. Using the paper to lift one layer, invert the cake and place it paper-side up on a large tray. Carefully peel off the paper. Spread with a thin layer of the raspberry jam.

8. Set a second layer paper-side up on top of the first. Remove the paper and spread the cake with the apricot jam.

9. Place the remaining layer paper-side up on top. Peel off the paper. With a large heavy knife and a ruler as a guide, trim the edges of the cake to make the layers straight and even all around.

10. Bring about 2 inches of water to a simmer in the bottom half of a double boiler or a small saucepan. Place the chocolate chips in the top half of the double boiler or in a small heatproof bowl that fits comfortably over the saucepan. Place the bowl over the simmering water. Let stand uncovered until the chocolate is softened. Stir until smooth. Pour the melted chocolate on top of the cake layers and spread it smooth with a spatula. Refrigerate until the chocolate is just beginning to set, about 30 minutes. (Don't let it get too hard, or it will crack when you cut it.)

11. Remove the cake from the refrigerator. Using a ruler or other straight edge as a guide, cut the cake lengthwise into 6 strips by first cutting it into thirds, then cutting each third in half. Cut crosswise into 5 strips. Chill the cut cake in the pan in the refrigerator until the chocolate is firm. Serve or transfer the cookies to an airtight container and store in the refrigerator. These keep well for several weeks.

Christmas Fig Cookies

Cuccidati

Makes 18 large cookies

I can't imagine Christmas without these cookies. For many Sicilians, making them is a family project. The women mix and roll the dough, while the men chop and grind the filling ingredients. The children decorate the filled cookies. They are traditionally cut into many fanciful shapes resembling birds, leaves, or flowers. Some families make dozens of them to give away to friends and neighbors.

Dough

2½ cups all-purpose flour

⅓ cup sugar

2 teaspoons baking powder

½ teaspoon salt

6 tablespoons unsalted butter

2 large eggs, at room temperature

1 teaspoon pure vanilla extract

Filling

2 cups moist dried figs, stems removed

½ cup raisins

1 cup walnuts, toasted and chopped

½ cup chopped semisweet chocolate (about 2 ounces)

⅓ cup honey

¼ cup orange juice

1 teaspoon orange zest

1 teaspoon ground cinnamon

⅛ teaspoon ground cloves

Assembly

1 egg yolk beaten with 1 teaspoon water

Colored candy sprinkles

1. Prepare the dough: In a large bowl, combine the flour, sugar, baking powder, and salt. Cut in the butter, using an electric mixer or pastry blender, until the mixture resembles coarse crumbs.

2. In a bowl, whisk the eggs and vanilla. Add the eggs to the dry ingredients, stirring with a wooden spoon until the dough is evenly moistened. If the dough is too dry, blend in a little cold water a few drops at a time.

3. Gather the dough into a ball and place it on a sheet of plastic wrap. Flatten it into a disk and wrap well. Refrigerate at least 1 hour or overnight.

4. Prepare the filling: In a food processor or meat grinder, grind the figs, raisins, and nuts until coarsely chopped. Stir in the remaining ingredients. Cover and refrigerate if not using within the hour.

5. To assemble the pastries, preheat the oven to 375°F. Grease two large baking sheets.

6. Cut the dough into 6 pieces. On a lightly floured surface, roll each piece into a log about 4 inches long.

7. With a floured rolling pin, roll one log into a 9 × 5-inch rectangle. Trim the edges.

8. Spoon a ³/₄-inch strip of the filling lengthwise slightly to one side of the center of the rolled out dough. Fold one long side of the dough over to the other and press the edges together to seal. Cut the filled dough crosswise into 3 even pieces.

9. With a sharp knife, cut slits ³/₄-inch long at ¹/₂-inch intervals through the filling and dough. Curving them slightly to open the slits and reveal the fig filling, place the pastries one inch apart on the baking sheets.

10. Brush the pastry with the egg wash. Drizzle with candy sprinkles if desired. Repeat with the remaining ingredients.

11. Bake the cookies 20 to 25 minutes or until golden brown.

12. Cool the cookies on wire racks. Store in an airtight container in the refrigerator up to 1 month.

Almond Brittle

Croccante or Torrone

Makes 10 to 12 servings

Sicilians make these sweets with pine nuts, pistachios, or sesame seeds in place of the almonds. A lemon is perfect to smooth out the hot syrup.

Vegetable oil

2 cups sugar

¼ cup honey

2 cups almonds (10 ounces)

1 whole lemon, washed and dried

1. Brush a marble surface or a metal baking sheet with neutral-flavored vegetable oil.

2. In a medium saucepan, combine the sugar and honey. Cook over medium-low heat, stirring occasionally, until the sugar begins to melt, about 20 minutes. Bring to a simmer and cook without stirring 5 minutes more or until the syrup is clear.

3. Add the nuts and cook until the syrup is amber-colored, about 3 minutes. Carefully pour the hot syrup onto the prepared surface, using the lemon to smooth the nuts to a single layer. Let cool completely. When the brittle is cool and hard, after about 30 minutes, slide a thin metal spatula underneath it. Lift the brittle and break it into $1^{1}/_{2}$-inch pieces. Store in airtight containers at room temperature.

Sicilian Nut Rolls

Mostaccioli

Makes 64 cookies

At one time these cookies were made with mosto cotto, concentrated wine grape juice. Today's cooks use honey.

Dough

3 cups all-purpose flour

½ cup sugar

1 teaspoon salt

½ cup shortening

4 tablespoons (½ stick) unsalted butter, at room temperature

2 large eggs

2 to 3 tablespoons cold milk

Filling

1 cup toasted almonds

1 cup toasted walnuts

½ cup toasted and skinned hazelnuts

¼ cup sugar

¼ cup honey

2 teaspoons orange zest

¼ teaspoon ground cinnamon

Confectioner's sugar

1. In a large bowl, combine the flour, sugar, and salt. Cut in the shortening and butter until the mixture resembles coarse crumbs.

2. In a small bowl, whisk the eggs with two tablespoons of the milk. Add the mixture to the dry ingredients, stirring until the dough is evenly moistened. If needed, blend in a little more milk.

3. Gather the dough into a ball and place it on a sheet of plastic wrap. Flatten it into a disk and wrap well. Refrigerate 1 hour up to overnight.

4. Process the nuts and sugar in a food processor. Process until fine. Add the honey, zest, and cinnamon, and process until

blended. Preheat the oven to 350°F. Grease 2 large baking sheets.

5. Divide the dough into 4 pieces. Roll out one piece between two sheets of plastic wrap to form a square slightly larger than 8 inches. Trim the edges and cut the dough into 2-inch squares. Place a heaping teaspoon of the filling along one side of each square. Roll up the dough to enclose the filling completely. Place seam-side down on the baking pan. Repeat with the remaining dough and filling, placing the cookies 1 inch apart.

6. Bake 18 minutes or until the cookies are lightly browned. Transfer the cookies to wire racks to cool. Store in a tightly sealed container up to 2 weeks. Sprinkle with confectioner's sugar before serving.

Sponge Cake

Pan di Spagna

Makes two 8- or 9-inch layers

This classic and versatile Italian sponge cake works well with fillings such as fruit preserves, whipped cream, pastry cream, ice cream, or ricotta cream. The cake also freezes well, so it is convenient to have on hand for quick desserts.

Butter for the pan

6 large eggs, at room temperature

⅔ cup sugar

1½ teaspoons pure vanilla extract

1 cup sifted all-purpose flour

1. Place the rack in the center of the oven. Preheat the oven to 375°F. Butter two 8- or 9-inch layer cake pans. Line the bottom of the pans with circles of waxed paper or parchment paper. Butter the paper. Dust the pans with flour and tap out the excess.

2. In a large bowl with an electric mixer, begin beating the eggs on low speed. Slowly add the sugar, gradually increasing the mixer speed to high. Add the vanilla. Beat the eggs until thick and pale yellow, about 7 minutes.

3. Place the flour in a fine-mesh strainer. Shake about one-third of the flour over the egg mixture. Gradually and very gently fold in the flour with a rubber spatula. Repeat, adding the flour in 2 additions and folding it in until there are no streaks.

4. Spread the batter evenly in the prepared pans. Bake 20 to 25 minutes or until the cakes spring back when pressed lightly in the center and the top is lightly browned. Have ready 2 cooling racks. Cool the cakes 10 minutes in the pans on the wire racks.

5. Invert the cakes onto the racks and remove the pans. Carefully peel off the paper. Let cool completely. Serve immediately or cover with an inverted bowl and store at room temperature up to 2 days.

Citrus Sponge Cake

Torta di Agrumi

Serves 10 to 12

Olive oil gives this cake a distinctive flavor and texture. Use a mild olive oil or the flavor could be intrusive. Because it does not contain butter, milk, or other dairy products, this cake is good for people who cannot eat those foods.

This is a big cake, though it is very light and airy. To bake it, you will need a 10-inch tube pan with a removable bottom—the kind used for angel cakes.

A little bit of cream of tartar, available in the spice section of most supermarkets, helps to stabilize the egg whites in this large cake.

2¼ cups plain cake flour (not self-rising)

1 tablespoon baking powder

1 teaspoon salt

6 large eggs, separated, at room temperature

1¼ cups sugar

1½ teaspoons orange zest

1½ teaspoons grated lemon zest

¾ cup freshly squeezed orange juice

½ cup extra-virgin olive oil

1 teaspoon pure vanilla extract

¼ teaspoon cream of tartar

1. Place the oven rack in the lower third of the oven. Preheat the oven to 325°F. In a large bowl, sift together the flour, baking powder, and salt.

2. In a large bowl with an electric mixer, beat the egg yolks, 1 cup of the sugar, the orange and lemon zests, the orange juice, oil, and vanilla extract until smooth, about 5 minutes. With a rubber spatula, fold the liquid into the dry ingredients.

3. In another large bowl with clean beaters, beat the egg whites on medium speed until foamy. Gradually add the remaining ¹/₄ cup of sugar and the cream of tartar. Increase the speed to high. Beat until soft peaks form when the beaters are lifted, about 5 minutes. Fold the whites into the batter.

4. Scrape the batter into an ungreased 10-inch tube pan with a removable bottom. Bake 55 minutes or until the cake is golden brown and a toothpick inserted in the center comes out clean.

5. Place the pan upside down on a cooling rack and let the cake cool completely. Run a thin-blade knife around the inside of the pan to loosen the cake. Lift out the cake and the bottom of the pan. Slide the knife under the cake and remove the pan bottom. Serve immediately, or cover with an overturned bowl and store at room temperature up to 2 days.

Lemon Olive-Oil Cake

Torta di Limone

Makes 8 servings

A light, lemony cake from Puglia that is always a pleasure to have on hand.

1½ cups plain cake flour (not self-rising)

1½ teaspoons baking powder

½ teaspoon salt

3 large eggs, at room temperature

1 cup sugar

⅓ cup olive oil

1 teaspoon pure vanilla extract

1 teaspoon grated lemon zest

¼ cup freshly squeezed lemon juice

1. Place the rack in the lowest third of the oven. Preheat oven to 350°F. Grease a 9-inch springform pan.

2. In a large bowl, sift together the flour, baking powder, and salt.

3. Break the eggs into a large electric mixer bowl. Beat on medium speed until thick and pale yellow, about 5 minutes. Slowly add in the sugar and beat 3 minutes more. Slowly add the oil. Beat one minute more. Add the vanilla and lemon zest.

4. With a rubber spatula, fold in the dry ingredients in three additions, alternating with the lemon juice in two additions.

5. Scrape the batter into the prepared pan. Bake 35 to 40 minutes or until the cake is golden brown and springs back when pressed in the center.

6. Turn the pan upside down on a wire rack. Let cool completely. Run a knife around the outside rim and remove it. Serve immediately, or cover with an overturned bowl and store at room temperature up to 2 days.

Marble Cake

Torta Marmorata

Makes 8 to 10 servings

Breakfast is not given a lot of attention in Italy. Eggs and cereal are rarely eaten, and most Italians get by on coffee with toast or perhaps a plain cookie or two. Hotel breakfasts often overcompensate for foreign tastes with a lavish variety of cold meats, cheeses, fruit, eggs, yogurt, bread, and pastries. At one hotel in Venice, I spotted a magnificent marble cake, one of my personal favorite cakes, proudly displayed on a cake stand. It was heavenly with a cup of cappuccino, and I would have enjoyed it equally at teatime. The waiter told me the cake was delivered fresh daily from a local bakery where it was a specialty. This is my version, inspired by the one in Venice.

1½ cups plain cake flour (not self-rising)

1½ teaspoons baking powder

½ teaspoon salt

3 large eggs, at room temperature

1 cup sugar

⅓ cup vegetable oil

1 teaspoon pure vanilla extract

¼ teaspoon almond extract

½ cup milk

2 ounces bittersweet or semisweet chocolate, melted and cooled

1. Place the oven rack in the lowest third of the oven. Preheat the oven to 325°F. Grease and flour a 10-inch tube pan and tap out the excess flour.

2. In a large bowl, sift together the flour, baking powder, and salt.

3. In another large bowl, with an electric mixer, beat the eggs on medium speed until thick and pale yellow, about 5 minutes. Slowly beat in the sugar a tablespoon at a time. Continue beating 2 minutes more.

4. Gradually beat in the oil and extracts. Fold in the flour in 3 additions, alternately adding the milk in two additions.

5. Remove about 1½ cups of the batter and place it in a small bowl. Set aside. Scrape the remaining batter into the prepared pan.

6. Fold the melted chocolate into the reserved batter. Place large spoonfuls of the chocolate batter on top of the batter in the pan. To swirl the batter, hold a table knife with the tip down. Insert the knife blade down through batter, running it gently all around the pan at least 2 times.

7. Bake 40 minutes or until the cake is golden brown and a toothpick comes out clean when inserted in the center. Let cool on a rack 10 minutes.

8. Invert the cake onto the rack and remove the pan. Turn the cake right-side up on another rack. Let cool completely. Serve immediately, or cover with an inverted bowl and store at room temperature up to 2 days.

Rum Cake

Baba au Rhum

Makes 8 to 10 servings

According to a popular story, this cake was invented by a Polish king who found his babka, a Polish yeast cake, too dry and poured a glass of rum on it. His creation was named baba, after Ali Baba of the Arabian Nights. How it became popular in Naples is not certain, but it has been for some time.

Because it is leavened with yeast rather than baking powder, baba has a spongy texture, perfect for absorbing the rum syrup. Some versions are baked in miniature muffin pans, while others have a pastry cream filling. I like to serve this with strawberries and whipped cream on the side—not typical, but delicious, and makes a lovely presentation.

1 package (2½ teaspoons) active dry yeast or instant yeast

¼ cup warm milk (100° to 110°F)

6 large eggs

2⅔ cups all-purpose flour

3 tablespoons sugar

½ teaspoon salt

¾ cup (1½ sticks) unsalted butter, at room temperature

Syrup

2 cups sugar

2 cups water

2 (2-inch) strips lemon zest

¼ cup rum

1. Grease a 10-inch tube pan.

2. Sprinkle the yeast over the warm milk. Let stand until creamy, about 1 minute, then stir until dissolved.

3. In a large mixing bowl, with an electric mixer on medium speed, beat the eggs until foamy, about 1 minute. Beat in the flour, sugar, and salt. Add the yeast and butter and beat until well blended, about 2 minutes

4. Scrape the dough into the prepared pan. Cover with plastic wrap and let stand in a warm place 1 hour or until the dough has doubled in volume.

5. Place a rack in the center of the oven. Preheat the oven to 400°F. Bake the cake 30 minutes or until it is golden and a toothpick inserted in the center comes out clean.

6. Invert the cake onto a cooling rack. Remove the pan and let cool for 10 minutes.

7. To make the syrup, combine the sugar, water, and lemon zest in a medium saucepan. Bring the mixture to a boil and stir until the sugar is dissolved, about 2 minutes. Remove the lemon zest. Stir in the rum. Set aside $1/4$ cup of the syrup.

8. Return the cake to the pan. With a fork, poke holes all over the surface. Slowly spoon the syrup over the cake while both are still hot. Let cool completely in the pan.

9. Just before serving, invert the cake onto a serving plate Drizzle with the remaining syrup. Serve immediately. Store covered with an overturned bowl at room temperature up to 2 days.

Grandmother's Cake

Torta della Nonna

Makes 8 servings

I couldn't decide whether to include this recipe—called torta della nonna—with the tarts or with the cakes; however, because Tuscans call it a torta, I include it with the cakes. It consists of two layers of pastry filled with a thick pastry cream. I don't know whose grandmother invented it, but everyone loves her cake. There are many variations, some including lemon flavoring.

1 cup milk

3 large egg yolks

⅓ cup sugar

1½ teaspoons pure vanilla extract

2 tablespoons all-purpose flour

2 tablespoons orange liqueur or rum

Dough

1⅔ cup all-purpose flour

½ cup sugar

1 teaspoon baking powder

½ teaspoon salt

½ cup (1 stick) unsalted butter, at room temperature

1 large egg, lightly beaten

1 teaspoon pure vanilla extract

1 egg yolk beaten with 1 teaspoon water, for egg wash

2 tablespoons pine nuts

Confectioner's sugar

1. In a medium saucepan, heat the milk over low heat until bubbles form around the edges. Remove from the heat.

2. In a medium bowl, whisk the egg yolks, sugar, and vanilla until pale yellow, about 5 minutes. Whisk in the flour. Gradually add the hot milk, whisking constantly. Transfer the mixture to the saucepan and cook over medium heat, stirring constantly, until boiling. Reduce the heat and simmer for 1 minute. Scrape the mixture into a bowl. Stir in the liqueur. Place a piece of plastic

wrap directly on the surface of the custard to prevent a skin from forming. Refrigerate 1 hour up to overnight.

3. Place the rack in the center of the oven. Preheat the oven to 350°F. Grease a 9 × 2-inch round cake pan.

4. Prepare the dough: In a large bowl, stir together the flour, sugar, baking powder, and salt. With a pastry blender, cut in the butter until the mixture resembles coarse crumbs. Add the egg and vanilla and stir until a dough forms. Divide the dough in half.

5. Scatter half of the dough evenly in the bottom of the prepared pan. Press the dough into the bottom of the pan and $1/2$ inch up the sides. Spread the chilled custard over the center of the dough, leaving a 1-inch border around the edge.

6. On a lightly floured surface, roll out the remaining dough to a $9 1/2$-inch circle. Place the dough over the filling. Press the edges of the dough together to seal. Brush the egg wash over the top of the cake. Sprinkle with the pine nuts. With a small knife, make several slits in the top to allow steam to escape.

7. Bake 35 to 40 minutes, or until golden brown on top. Let cool in the pan on a rack for 10 minutes.

8. Invert the cake onto the rack, then invert onto another rack to cool completely. Sprinkle with confectioner's sugar before serving. Serve immediately, or wrap the cake in plastic wrap and refrigerate up to 8 hours. Wrap and store in the refrigerator.

Apricot Almond Cake

Torta di Albicocche e Mandorle

Makes 8 servings

Apricots and almonds are very compatible flavors. If you can't find fresh apricots, substitute peaches or nectarines.

Topping

2/3 cup sugar

1/4 cup water

12 to 14 apricots or 6 to 8 peaches, halved, pitted, and cut into 1/4-inch-thick slices

Cake

1 cup all-purpose flour

1 teaspoon baking powder

1/2 teaspoon salt

1/2 cup almond paste

2 tablespoons unsalted butter

⅔ cup sugar

½ teaspoon pure vanilla extract

2 large eggs

⅔ cup milk

1. Prepare the topping: Place the sugar and water in a small heavy saucepan. Cook over medium heat, stirring occasionally, until the sugar is completely dissolved, about 3 minutes. When the mixture begins to boil, stop stirring and cook until the syrup starts to brown around the edges. Then gently swirl the pan over the heat until the syrup is an even golden brown, about 2 minutes more.

2. Protecting your hand with a pot holder, immediately pour the caramel into a 9 × 2-inch round cake pan. Tilt the pan to coat the bottom evenly. Let the caramel cool until set, about 5 minutes.

3. Place the oven rack in the center of the oven. Preheat the oven to 350°F. Arrange the sliced fruit, overlapping them slightly, in circles on top of the caramel.

4. Combine the flour, baking powder, and salt in a fine-mesh strainer set over a piece of wax paper. Sift the dry ingredients onto the paper.

5. In a large electric mixer bowl, beat the almond paste, butter, sugar, and vanilla until fluffy, about 4 minutes. Beat in the eggs one at a time, scraping the side of the bowl. Continue beating until smooth and well blended, about 4 minutes more.

6. With the mixer on low speed, stir in $1/3$ of the flour mixture. Add $1/3$ of the milk. Add the remaining flour mixture and milk in two more additions in the same way, ending with the flour. Stir just until smooth.

7. Pour the batter over the fruit. Bake 40 to 45 minutes or until the cake is golden and a toothpick inserted in the center comes out clean.

8. Let the cake cool in the pan on a wire rack 10 minutes. Run a thin metal spatula around the inside of the pan. Invert the cake onto a serving plate (the fruit will be on top) and let cool completely before serving. Serve immediately, or cover with an inverted bowl and store at room temperature up to 24 hours.

Summer Fruit Torte

Torta dell'Estate

Makes 8 servings

Soft stone fruits such as plums, apricots, peaches, and nectarines are ideal for this torte. Try making it with a combination of fruits.

12 to 16 prune plums or apricots, or 6 medium peaches or nectarines, halved, pitted, and cut into ½-inch slices

1 cup all-purpose flour

1 teaspoon baking powder

½ teaspoon salt

½ cup (1 stick) unsalted butter, at room temperature

⅔ cup plus 2 tablespoons sugar

1 large egg

1 teaspoon grated lemon zest

1 teaspoon pure vanilla extract

Confectioner's sugar

1. Place the rack in the center of the oven. Preheat the oven to 350°F. Grease a 9-inch springform pan.

2. In a large bowl, mix together the flour, baking powder, and salt.

3. In another large bowl, beat the butter with $2/3$ cup of the sugar until light and fluffy, about 3 minutes. Beat in the egg, lemon zest, and vanilla until smooth. Add the dry ingredients and stir just until blended, about 1 minute more.

4. Scrape the batter into the prepared pan. Arrange the fruit, overlapping it slightly, on top in concentric circles. Sprinkle with the remaining 2 tablespoons of sugar.

5. Bake 45 to 50 minutes or until the cake is golden brown and a toothpick inserted in the center comes out clean.

6. Let the cake cool in the pan on a wire rack 10 minutes, then remove the rim of the pan. Let the cake cool completely. Sprinkle with confectioner's sugar before serving. Serve immediately, or cover with an overturned bowl and store at room temperature up to 24 hours.

Autumn Fruit Torte

Torta del Autunno

Makes 8 servings

Apples, pears, figs, or plums are good in this simple cake. The batter forms a top layer that does not quite cover the fruit, allowing it to peek through the surface of the cake. I like to serve it slightly warm.

1½ cups all-purpose flour

1 teaspoon baking powder

½ teaspoon salt

2 large eggs

1 cup sugar

1 teaspoon pure vanilla extract

4 tablespoons unsalted butter, melted and cooled

2 medium apples or pears, peeled, cored, and sliced into thin wedges

Confectioner's sugar

1. Place the rack in the center of the oven. Preheat the oven to 350°F. Grease and flour a 9-inch springform cake pan. Tap out the excess flour.

2. In a bowl, stir together the flour, baking powder, and salt.

3. In a large bowl, beat the eggs with the sugar and vanilla until blended, about 2 minutes. Beat in the butter. Stir in the flour mixture until just blended, about 1 minute more.

4. Spread half of the batter in the prepared pan. Cover with the fruits. Drop the remaining batter on top by spoonfuls. Spread the batter evenly over the fruits. The layer will be thin. Don't be concerned if the fruit is not completely covered.

5. Bake 30 to 35 minutes or until the cake is golden brown and a toothpick inserted in the center comes out clean.

6. Let the cake cool 10 minutes in the pan on a wire rack. Remove the rim of the pan. Cool the cake completely on the rack. Serve warm or at room temperature with a sprinkle of confectioner's sugar. Store covered with a large inverted bowl at room temperature up to 24 hours.

Polenta and Pear Cake

Dolce di Polenta

Makes 8 servings

Yellow cornmeal adds a pleasant texture and warm golden color to this rustic cake from the Veneto.

1 cup all-purpose flour

⅓ cup finely ground yellow cornmeal

1 teaspoon baking powder

½ teaspoon salt

¾ cup (1½ sticks) unsalted butter, softened

¾ cup plus 2 tablespoons sugar

1 teaspoon pure vanilla extract

½ teaspoon grated lemon zest

2 large eggs

⅓ cup milk

1 large ripe pear, cored and thinly sliced

1. Place a rack in the center of the oven. Preheat the oven to 350°F. Grease and flour a 9-inch springform pan. Tap out the excess flour.

2. In a large bowl, sift together the flour, cornmeal, baking powder, and salt.

3. In a large bowl with an electric mixer, beat the butter, gradually adding $3/4$ cup of the sugar until light and fluffy, about 3 minutes. Beat in the vanilla and lemon zest. Beat in the eggs one at time, scraping the sides of the bowl. On low speed, stir in half of the dry ingredients. Add the milk. Stir in the remaining dry ingredients just until smooth, about 1 minute.

4. Spread the batter in the prepared pan. Arrange the pear slices on top, overlapping them slightly. Sprinkle the pear with the remaining 2 tablespoons of sugar.

5. Bake 45 minutes or until the cake is golden brown and a toothpick inserted in the center comes out clean.

6. Cool the cake in the pan 10 minutes on a wire rack. Remove the pan rim and cool the cake completely on the rack. Serve

immediately, or cover with a large inverted bowl and store at room temperature up to 24 hours.

www.ingramcontent.com/pod-product-compliance
Lightning Source LLC
Chambersburg PA
CBHW071820080526
44589CB00012B/867